# Table of Contents

# Practice Test #1

## Practice Questions

1. A patient has been admitted to the hospital for status epilepticus. The patient is currently postictal. Which of the following is the most important nursing consideration for managing the patient?
    a. Obtain an electrocardiogram.
    b. Insert a central line.
    c. Prepare the patient for a lumbar puncture.
    d. Maintain an airway.

2. A young child is brought into the hospital for recurrent staring episodes while at school. What is the most likely etiology for her symptoms?
    a. Simple partial seizure.
    b. Pseudoseizure.
    c. Petit mal seizure.
    d. Grand mal seizure.

3. An 85-year-old woman presents to the emergency department with facial droop, dysarthria, and unilateral weakness that started 6 hours prior to arrival. Her medical history includes hypertension and gallbladder surgery last week. Her blood pressure in the emergency department is 165/85. Which of the following is an absolute contraindication for administering tissue plasminogen activator (tPA)?
    a. Age.
    b. Symptom onset.
    c. Blood pressure.
    d. Recent abdominal surgery.

4. What nutritional advice is best for a patient who will be discharged at home on warfarin (Coumadin) to prevent recurrence of embolic stroke?
    a. Green leafy vegetables are OK to eat in moderation.
    b. Iron supplements are advised.
    c. Take a vitamin K supplement because warfarin inhibits vitamin K.
    d. Do not drink more than 2 glasses of wine per week.

5. A patient is about to undergo a lumbar puncture at bedside. What is the most important part of the nursing preparation?
    a. Have the patient lie flat.
    b. Check coagulation panel and platelet count.
    c. Make sure the patient has central venous access.
    d. Have patient use bathroom prior to procedure .

6. A patient has an external ventricular drain. The intracranial pressure (ICP) ranges from 25 to 30 mm Hg. Which of the following signs/symptoms would not be consistent with these ICPs?
    a. Tachycardia.
    b. Fixed pupils.
    c. Bradycardia.
    d. Irregular respirations.

7. What is the best dietary advice to give a patient diagnosed with myasthenia gravis?
    a. Eat 6 small meals per day.
    b. Maintain a liquid-only diet .
    c. Eat primarily in the mornings when energy level is highest.
    d. See a nutritionist weekly to monitor feedings.

8. Which of the following is the most accurate diagnostic test for Chiari malformation?
    a. PET scan.
    b. CT scan.
    c. MRI.
    d. Ultrasound.

9. Which position is a patient advised to maintain to minimize symptoms following a lumbar puncture?
    a. Prone.
    b. Reverse Trendelenburg.
    c. Sitting up.
    d. Fowler's.

10. A patient with an external ventricular drain (EVD) has an ICP of 30 mm Hg. The output of the drain is very sluggish when it is opened. What is the next step?
    a. Flush the drain proximally.
    b. Continue to monitor the ICP.
    c. Flush the drain distally.
    d. Call the attending/resident.

11. A patient's Tinetti score is 19 prior to a lumbar puncture. After the lumbar puncture, the Tinetti score improves to 28. What is the most likely diagnosis?
    a. Acute disseminating encephalomyelitis.
    b. Bacterial meningitis.
    c. Normal pressure hydrocephalus.
    d. Posterior reversible encephalopathy syndrome.

12. A patient has had a stroke involving the limbic system. What type of deficit is most likely to result?
    a. Visual impairment.
    b. Flat affect.
    c. Fluent aphasia.
    d. Impulsive inhibition difficulty.

13. A patient who has had a stroke is going to be discharged with aspirin (Ecotrin) and ticagrelor (Brilinta). Which of the following side effects of these medications should the family be educated about?
    a. Bleeding.
    b. Nystagmus.
    c. Tardive dyskinesia.
    d. Ataxia.

14. All of the following methods are used to decrease intracranial pressure EXCEPT:
    a. hypotonic intravenous fluids.
    b. diuretics.
    c. sedation.
    d. hyperventilation.

15. Which of the following interventions would likely be needed in a patient with end-stage Creutzfeldt-Jakob disease?
    a. Percutaneous endoscopic gastrostomy (PEG) tube.
    b. Lumbar puncture.
    c. Ventricular peritoneal shunt.
    d. Anti-inflammatory medications.

16. The nurse is assessing the motor function of an unconscious patient. Which of the following can be used to test the patient's peripheral response to pain?
    a. Using a reflex hammer on the patella.
    b. Applying nailbed pressure.
    c. Squeezing of the sternocleidomastoid muscle.
    d. Dropping saline in the patient's eyes.

17. A nurse is treating a patient with pneumococcal meningitis. Which of the following are the most important measures to prevent the spread of the disease?
    a. Handwashing, booties, and gown.
    b. Face mask, booties, and gown.
    c. Booties, gown, and gloves.
    d. Face mask, gown, and gloves.

18. A patient suddenly develops extremity tremors, drooling, and eye-rolling. The episode resolves spontaneously and afterward the patient is confused and lethargic. What type of seizure did this patient most likely experience?
    a. Grand mal seizure.
    b. Petit mal seizure.
    c. Absence seizure.
    d. Simple partial seizure.

19. An incarcerated patient with a history of HIV develops lethargy, anorexia, vomiting, and high-grade fever. On physical exam the patient has a positive Brudzinski sign. Which of the following tests would not be used to confirm the diagnosis?
    a. Lumbar puncture.
    b. Blood cultures.
    c. CT scan of the abdomen and pelvis.
    d. Erythrocyte sedimentation rate.

20. What is the common primary brain tumor in American adults?
    a. Pituitary adenoma.
    b. Glioblastoma multiforme.
    c. Acoustic neuroma.
    d. Wilms tumor.

21. A 71-year-old man is involved in a car accident. He denies complaints but undergoes an MRI of the brain, which reveals a 3 mm meningioma. What is the best course of initial treatment?
    a. Schedule the patient for a craniotomy.
    b. Schedule the patient for radiation.
    c. Follow-up imaging of the brain.
    d. Obtain a CT scan of the chest, abdomen, and pelvis.

22. A patient is diagnosed with a malignant lesion in the frontal cortex. Which of the following is most likely to be affected?
    a. Sleep/wake cycles.
    b. Memory.
    c. Behavior inhibition.
    d. Fine motor movements.

23. Which medication is the first-line therapy in treating absence seizures?
    a. Ethosuximide (Zarontin).
    b. Phenytoin (Dilantin).
    c. Levetiracetam (Keppra).
    d. Lacosamide (Vimpat).

24. A 44-year-old woman arrives in the emergency department after being involved in a high-speed motor vehicle accident. A CT scan of the head reveals a convex hypodensity in the right parietal cortex. What is the most likely diagnosis?
    a. Epidural hematoma.
    b. Subarachnoid hemorrhage.
    c. Subdural hematoma.
    d. Hemorrhagic contusion.

25. A patient status post hemicraniectomy is being discharged to a rehabilitation center. The patient's spouse asks how often he should be wearing his craniectomy helmet. What is the most appropriate response?
    a. He does not need to wear it while at rehab.
    b. He should wear it all of the time.
    c. He should wear it only when unsupervised.
    d. He should wear it only when out of bed.

26. A patient with an EVD has developed a steadily increasing ICP. Which of the following medications should the nurse expect to be given to this patient?
    a. Hydralazine.
    b. Furosemide (Lasix).
    c. Hydrochlorothiazide (Microzide).
    d. Mannitol (Osmitrol).

27. A patient admitted for a stroke had been given tissue plasminogen activator (tPA) 10 hours ago. The patient has failed his swallow evaluation and is due for ticagrelor (Brilinta). What should the nurse do?

    a. Place a nasogastric tube and give the medications.
    b. Crush the medications and give it to him with applesauce.
    c. Hold the dose for another 14 hours.
    d. Give ticagrelor to the patient rectally.

28. A patient admitted for a traumatic brain injury has failed his swallow evaluation for 5 consecutive days. Which of the following should the nurse suggest to the medical team in regard to the patient's nutrition?

    a. Pureed diet.
    b. Liquid diet.
    c. Tube feeds.
    d. Total parenteral nutrition.

29. A patient on warfarin (Coumadin) complains of headache for the past several days after accidentally striking his head against a car door. A CT scan reveals bilateral concave hypodensities in the temporal lobes. What is the most likely  diagnosis?

    a. Hemorrhagic contusion.
    b. Subdural hematoma.
    c. Epidural hematoma.
    d. Diffuse axonal injury.

30. A patient is admitted with an aneurysmal subarachnoid hemorrhage. Which of the following treatment modalities are the mainstays of therapy?

    a. Hypertension, hemodilution, hypervolemia.
    b. Hypercoagulability, hypertension, hyperglycemia.
    c. Hypertension, hemodilution, hypovolemia.
    d. Hypotension, hemodilution, hypovolemia.

31. A patient complains of chronic back pain that has worsened over the past several weeks. An x-ray shows straightening of the thoracic spine with loss of normal curvature and exaggerated inward curvature of the lumbar spine. What is the most likely diagnosis?

    a. Lordosis.
    b. Spondylolisthesis.
    c. Kyphosis.
    d. Scoliosis.

32. A patient is being discharged from the hospital after being diagnosed and treated for trigeminal neuralgia. Which of the following is not an appropriate recommendation for the nurse to give to the patient?

    a. Shaving may precipitate pain.
    b. Eating soft foods may prevent symptoms.
    c. Chewing gum may help symptoms.
    d. Drinking room temperature drinks may help prevent pain.

33. A patient with a traumatic brain injury on a mechanical ventilator has a mean arterial pressure (MAP) of 82 and a cerebral perfusion pressure (CPP) of 26. Which of the following interventions would be most appropriate in this patient?
    a. Decreasing the fractured inspired oxygen ($FiO_2$).
    b. Decreasing the respiratory rate.
    c. Increasing the positive end-expiratory pressure (PEEP).
    d. Increasing the respiratory rate.

34. A patient is admitted to the hospital for an exacerbation of her Meniere disease. What is the most appropriate diet for this patient to help prevent exacerbation of her symptoms?
    a. Lactose free.
    b. Low sodium.
    c. Gluten free.
    d. Low sugar.

35. What is the most common cause of an arteriovenous malformation (AVM)?
    a. Tobacco abuse.
    b. Idiopathic.
    c. Obesity.
    d. Hypertension.

36. A 16-year-old patient is brought to the clinic by his parents complaining of progressive severe middle and lower back pain. His parents blame his symptoms on his poor posture. Imaging reveals a significant outward curvature of the thoracic spine. Which of the following is the most likely diagnosis?
    a. Pott disease
    b. Scheuermann disease
    c. Amyotrophic lateral sclerosis (ALS)
    d. Neurofibromatosis

37. A 21-year-old patient with no past medical history arrives at the hospital with a suspected carotid dissection. Which of the following is the most important lab that needs to be sent prior to arteriography?
    a. Erythrocyte sedimentation rate (ESR).
    b. Liver function tests (LFTs).
    c. Basic metabolic panel (BMP).
    d. Complete blood cell count (CBC).

38. A patient has been brought to the hospital following an assault. A CT scan of the head is negative and the patient is eventually discharged. Two weeks later the patient returns with nausea, vomiting, and lethargy. A CT of the head reveals bilateral concave hypodensities in the parietal lobes. What is the most likely diagnosis?
    a. Subacute epidural hematomas.
    b. Acute subdural hematomas.
    c. Chronic subdural hematomas.
    d. Subacute subdural hematomas.

39. A patient is diagnosed with a 2 mm posterior communicating artery unruptured aneurysm. Which of the following in the most appropriate interventions?
    a. Order imaging of the chest and abdomen.
    b. No intervention.
    c. Aneurysm clip or coil.
    d. Repeat imaging in 6 months.

40. A patient with suspected hypoxic brain injury following a traumatic event has been declining in her neurological exam. She does not take spontaneous breaths on the ventilator or respond to painful stimuli, and her pupils do not react to light. Which of the following is appropriate if the family refuses a palliative care consult?
    a. Initiate brain death protocol.
    b. Call palliative care anyway.
    c. Remove the patient from the ventilator.
    d. Continue to monitor the patient.

41. An 89-year-old patient with lung cancer with metastases to the bone, liver, and brain is having significant difficulty eating. The speech therapist is recommending that a percutaneous endoscopic gastrostomy (PEG) tube be placed in order to maintain adequate nutrition. The patient is neurologically intact and is refusing the feeding tube. The patient is requesting hospice placement. The patient's spouse wants a PEG tube placed. Which of the following is the most appropriate intervention?
    a. Order a surgery consult for PEG placement.
    b. Continue daily dysphagia evaluations.
    c. Order a palliative care consult.
    d. Order a calorie count.

42. A 5-year-old child is admitted for worsening headaches and seizure. This patient has no past medical history. MRI of the brain reveals a mass in the fourth ventricle. Which of the following is the most likely diagnosis?
    a. Acoustic neuroma.
    b. Ependymoma.
    c. Vestibular schwannoma.
    d. Brainstem glioma.

43. A young patient presents with café au lait spots, bony deformities, short stature, and macrocephaly. Which of the following is the most appropriate intervention for this child?
    a. Referral to a dermatologist.
    b. Referral to a physical therapist.
    c. Referral to an audiologist.
    d. Referral to a gastroenterologist.

44. A patient has been diagnosed with amyotrophic lateral sclerosis (ALS). The patient has bilateral muscle atrophy and weakness, but can still perform most activities of daily life with assistance. He and his wife inquire about the goals of medical care. What is the best response?
    a. The goal is to keep the patient mobile for as long as possible.
    b. The goal is to treat the patient and halt the progression of symptoms.
    c. The goal is treat the disease and reverse the symptoms.
    d. The goal is monitor the patient for possible progression.

45. A patient who had previously sustained multiple facial and sinus fractures several weeks ago now presents with fever, headache, nausea, and vomiting. MRI reveals a ring-enhancing mass. What is the most likely diagnosis?
   a. Subarachnoid hemorrhage.
   b. Epidural hematoma.
   c. Meningioma.
   d. Brain abscess.

46. A patient develops bilateral lower extremity weakness that has spread to her upper extremities over the past several days. She is also complaining of "pins and needles" sensation in her extremities. She has no significant past medical history other than having an upper respiratory infection several weeks ago. What is the most likely treatment?
   a. Pyridostigmine (Regonol).
   b. Aspirin (Ecotrin).
   c. Plasmapheresis.
   d. Antibiotics.

47. Which of the following is not a likely sign of vertebral artery dissection?
   a. Transient ischemic attack (TIA).
   b. Neck pain.
   c. Frontal headache.
   d. Visual loss.

48. A patient who had been on aspirin (Ecotrin) and clopidogrel (Plavix) for prior transient ischemic attacks has another transient ischemic attack. During his workup, his carotid Doppler ultrasound reveals 50 percent stenosis of his right carotid artery. What is the next step in management?
   a. Change aspirin to ticagrelor.
   b. Carotid endarterectomy.
   c. Administration of tPA.
   d. Change clopidogrel to warfarin.

49. What is the most likely complication of an intraventricular hemorrhage?
   a. Blindness.
   b. Abscess.
   c. Hydrocephalus.
   d. Seizure.

50. Which of the following is the most common cause for lacunar strokes?
   a. Hypertension.
   b. Alcohol abuse.
   c. Hyperlipidemia.
   d. Obesity.

51. A patient who has had a stroke is being discharged home today. The patient's wife is concerned about caring for her husband at home. Which of the following is not an appropriate response to the patient's wife?
    a. Advise her to let him resume activity as tolerated.
    b. Advise her to make a daily to-do list.
    c. Advise bedrest except for bathing or toileting.
    d. Advise to call 911 if there is any change in his behavior.

52. Which of the following two medications should not be taken together?
    a. Aspirin (Ecotrin) and atorvastatin (Lipitor).
    b. Ticagrelor (Brilinta) and warfarin (Coumadin).
    c. Aspirin (Ecotrin) and clopidogrel (Plavix).
    d. Esomeprazole (Nexium) and clopidogrel (Plavix).

53. Which of the following does not need to be avoided when taking warfarin?
    a. Kale.
    b. Ginger.
    c. Alcohol.
    d. Iceberg lettuce.

54. A 1-year-old child with no significant past medical history experiences a febrile seizure. Which of the following is not a true statement regarding febrile seizures?
    a. A febrile seizure is different than epilepsy.
    b. Febrile seizures are relative common in young children.
    c. Most febrile seizures are harmless.
    d. Anticonvulsants are recommended to prevent future episodes.

55. A patient is in the ICU for an intracerebral hemorrhage. Which of the following IV fluids is contraindicated in this patient?
    a. D5W.
    b. Lactated Ringer's.
    c. Normal saline.
    d. Sodium chloride 3%.

56. A patient remains in a persistent vegetative state following a high-speed car collision. CT scans have shown mild cerebral edema but no other abnormality. MRI of the brain reveals several punctuate hypodensities in addition to cerebral edema. What is the most likely diagnosis?
    a. Subdural hematoma.
    b. Diffuse axonal injury.
    c. Multiple sclerosis.
    d. Subarachnoid hemorrhage.

57. Which of the following is consistent with Brown–Séquard syndrome?
    a. Loss of proprioception on the ipsilateral side as the injury
    b. Loss of temperature sensation on the ipsilateral side as the injury
    c. Loss of proprioception on the contralateral side as the injury
    d. Babinski sign contralateral to the side as the injury

58. Which of the following is a rare etiology of spondylolisthesis?
   a. Isthmic.
   b. Degenerative disease.
   c. Trauma.
   d. Pathologic.

59. Which of the following injuries is most likely to need a percutaneous gastrostomy (PEG) tube?
   a. C2.
   b. C7.
   c. T2.
   d. T7.

60. A patient has a traumatic brain injury and a skull fracture following an assault. The nurse noted a halo sign on his sheets next to his right ear. Which bone did the patient most likely fracture?
   a. Frontal.
   b. Temporal.
   c. Parietal.
   d. Occipital.

61. Which of the following conditions increases the risk of cerebrovascular accident fourfold?
   a. Morbid obesity.
   b. Hypertension.
   c. Cocaine abuse.
   d. Atrial fibrillation.

62. An incidental hemangioblastoma is found on imaging. What is the most appropriate intervention?
   a. Chemotherapy.
   b. Radiation.
   c. Serial imaging.
   d. Surgical excision.

63. Which following most likely metastasize to the brain?
   a. Renal cell carcinoma.
   b. Lymphoma.
   c. Colorectal cancer.
   d. Pancreatic cancer.

64. A patient involved in a diving accident has an injury to his spine. He has impaired function of his arms requiring assistance with oral feeds. He is paraplegic and can operate a motorized wheelchair. He is able to breathe on his own. He is incontinent and requires an indwelling catheter. Which of the following levels is most likely affected?
   a. C2.
   b. C7.
   c. T2.
   d. T7.

65. Following the administration of a vaccine 1 week prior, an otherwise healthy child develops headache, nausea, vomiting, confusion, and visual disturbances. After administration of steroids, the patient's condition gradually improves. What is the most likely diagnosis?
    a. Acute disseminating encephalomyelitis (ADEM).
    b. Chronic inflammatory demyelinating polyneuropathy (CIDP).
    c. Myasthenia gravis (MG).
    d. Amyotrophic lateral sclerosis (ALS).

66. A patient presents with a gradually worsening tremor that started in his right arm and traveled to his right leg. He remained conscious throughout the entire episode and was awake and alert following the episode. What type of seizure did he experience?
    a. Simple partial seizure.
    b. Complex partial seizure.
    c. Petit mal seizure.
    d. Grand mal seizure.

67. Which of the following is not true regarding posterior reversible encephalopathy syndrome (PRES)?
    a. Malignant hypertension may cause PRES.
    b. If left untreated, it can cause hydrocephalus.
    c. CT scan is the best diagnostic scan.
    d. Seizures are the most common presenting symptom.

68. A patient is trying to get pregnant and inquires how to help prevent her unborn child from developing spina bifida. What is the most appropriate response?
    a. Having 1 or 2 glasses of red wine a night.
    b. Eating a low-sugar diet.
    c. Drinking 3 glasses of milk per day.
    d. Eating several oranges daily.

69. Which of the following statements regarding acute disseminated encephalomyelitis (ADEM) and multiple sclerosis (MS) are false?
    a. Steroids are used in the medical care of both MS and ADEM.
    b. ADEM primarily occurs in young adults.
    c. ADEM is an inflammatory demyelinating condition.
    d. MS is a chronic relapsing and remitting disease.

70. An obese female with a known history of cocaine abuse is admitted for an acute ischemic stroke. The patient has a known history of sickle cell disease and hypertension. How many risk factors for stroke does this patient have?
    a. Two.
    b. Three.
    c. Four.
    d. Five.

71. A 70-year-old African American man with a history of tobacco abuse and diabetes presents to the ER with a right facial droop. He is diagnosed with an acute lacunar infarction and admitted. During his workup he is found to have a blood pressure of 178/98. His hemoglobin A1c is 9.2. His low-density lipoprotein (LDL) is 165. How many non–modifiable risk factors does this patient have?
    a. Two.
    b. Three.
    c. Five.
    d. Six.

72. Which test should be ordered for suspected cryptococcal meningitis?
    a. Western blot.
    b. India ink.
    c. Rapid plasma reagin (RPR).
    d. Monospot test.

73. A patient with suspected meningitis has undergone a lumbar puncture. Which of the following CSF results are most consistent with a viral etiology?
    a. Purulent CSF, high WBC count, elevated protein level.
    b. Clear CSF, high WBC count, elevated protein level.
    c. Clear CSF, normal WBC count, normal protein level.
    d. Purulent CSF, high WBC count, elevated protein level.

74. When educating a patient about the warning signs of stroke, which of the following best describes the most common symptoms?
    a. Loss of memory, ataxia, urinary incontinence.
    b. Hearing loss, facial weakness, headache.
    c. Facial droop, asymmetric weakness, dysarthria.
    d. Ataxia, resting tremor, muscle rigidity.

75. A patient is placed on warfarin after an embolic stroke. The patient's international normalized ratio (INR) is 1.5. The current dosage is 2 mg per day. What should the provider do regarding the dosage?
    a. Increase the dosage to 4 mg per day.
    b. Increase the dosage to 8 mg per day.
    c. Maintain the same dosage.
    d. Decrease the dosage to 1 mg per day.

76. Which one of these evaluations should be assessed first in a patient who recently had a stroke?
    a. Skin assessment.
    b. Coping evaluation.
    c. Ability to void.
    d. Swallow evaluation.

77. A patient with an external ventricular drain (EVD) has intracranial pressures (ICPs) ranging from 25 to 30 mmHg. There is no change in the neurological exam. Which of the following is the most appropriate intervention?
    a. No intervention; monitor the patient.
    b. Raise the head of bed to 30 degrees.
    c. Flush the EVD.
    d. Administer mannitol (Osmitrol).

78. A patient is being discharged home with his family after being hospitalized for a stroke. Which of the following statements indicate the family needs further instruction?
    a. My family member's symptoms will resolve in a few months.
    b. If my family member develops new symptoms I will call 911.
    c. I will assist as needed with activities of daily life.
    d. I can expect that my family member and I may get frustrated.

79. The following interventions are most likely to promote maximum self-care for a patient recovering from a traumatic brain injury, EXCEPT:
    a. allow the patient to ambulate without assistance to promote strength.
    b. provide adaptive equipment as indicated.
    c. educate patient on risks of repeat stroke.
    d. encourage participation in activities of daily living.

80. A nurse enters a patient's room following a cardiac catheterization and notes that the patient is slurring. Which of the following actions should be done last?
    a. Assess vital signs.
    b. Do a full neurological assessment.
    c. Order a CT scan of the brain.
    d. Perform a dysphagia evaluation.

81. Which of the following interventions is not appropriate for treating a patient with a chronic subdural hematoma?
    a. Physical therapy evaluation.
    b. Serial neurologic exams.
    c. Give an anticonvulsant drug for prophylaxis.
    d. Cognitive assessment.

82. Which of the following is the most common traumatic brain injury?
    a. Subdural hematoma.
    b. Subarachnoid hemorrhage.
    c. Concussion.
    d. Diffuse axonal injury.

83. A 33-year-old woman has a headache, slurred speech, coordination difficulties, and visual changes. She undergoes an MRI of the brain, which shows nonspecific white matter lesions consistent with plaque formation. Which of the following is the most appropriate treatment?
    a. Antibiotics.
    b. Steroids.
    c. Antiplatelet therapy.
    d. Nonsteroidal anti-inflammatory drugs (NSAIDs).

84. What is the primary neurotransmitter affected in Parkinson disease?
    a. Epinephrine.
    b. Dopamine.
    c. Serotonin.
    d. Histamine.

85. Which of the following best describes the etiology for Creutzfeldt–Jakob disease?
    a. Prions.
    b. Autoimmune.
    c. Bacteria.
    d. Unknown.

86. Which of the following diseases would find Lewy bodies on brain biopsy?
    a. Parkinson disease.
    b. Myasthenia gravis.
    c. Multiple sclerosis.
    d. Craniopharyngioma.

87. A patient is brought to the emergency department for altered mental status. She has a bag of medications with her, but cannot recall her medical issues. One of the pill bottles is carbidopa–levodopa (Sinemet). Which medical condition does she have?
    a. Creutzfeldt–Jakob disease.
    b. Myasthenia gravis.
    c. Multiple sclerosis.
    d. Parkinson disease.

88. A patient's wife has just been told that her husband, who has been on hospice care for stage IV glioma, just died. She originally denied that he could be dead. She then became angry and started to blame his medical providers. Which of the following is not an appropriate action?
    a. Calling the police.
    b. Calling a social worker.
    c. Calling a grief counselor.
    d. Calling a psychiatrist.

89. A 29-year-old man had a new–onset seizure after being involved in an assault. He is postictal, but is able to protect his own airway. Which of the following medications is the best initial medication to administer?
    a. Ethosuximide (Zarontin).
    b. Phenytoin (Dilantin).
    c. Levetiracetam (Keppra).
    d. Pentobarbital (Nembutal).

90. Which of the following is true regarding craniopharyngiomas?
    a. They occur in the brainstem.
    b. They are benign tumors.
    c. They primarily occur in children.
    d. There are no known risk factors.

91. A woman whose husband has been diagnosed with Huntington disease inquires how the disease is acquired. Which of the following responses is correct?
    a. Autosomal recessive.
    b. Idiopathic.
    c. Autosomal dominant.
    d. X–linked recessive.

92. A patient presents with progressively worsening personality changes and emotional issues. On physical exam the patient has a left facial droop and left-sided weakness. An MRI of the brain reveals a glioma. Where is the most likely location of the mass?
    a. Left frontal cortex.
    b. Left temporal cortex.
    c. Right frontal cortex.
    d. Right temporal cortex.

93. A patient is admitted with progressive neurological changes and blindness. A lumbar puncture is performed and the culture reveals *Treponema pallidum.* Which of the following is the most appropriate treatment?
    a. Penicillin (Nafcillin).
    b. Acyclovir (Zorivax).
    c. Amphotericin B (Fungizone).
    d. Sulfamethoxazole/Trimethoprim (Bactrim).

94. A patient has suspected aneurysmal subarachnoid hemorrhage, but the CT scan of the brain is negative. What is another test that can confirm the diagnosis?
    a. Skull series.
    b. Transcranial Doppler.
    c. MRI of the brain.
    d. Lumbar puncture.

95. A patient in the intensive care unit is admitted for a ruptured cerebral aneurysm. Which medication should be ordered to help prevent vasospasm?
    a. Metoprolol (Lopressor).
    b. Nimodipine (Nimotop).
    c. Carvedilol (Coreg).
    d. Candesartan (Atacand).

96. A 16-year-old female patient comes to the clinic with progressively worsening pedunculated masses over her entire body. She states that they are itching and painful. Several relatives have similar signs and symptoms. Which of the following is the most likely diagnosis?
    a. Ependymoma.
    b. Hemangioblastoma.
    c. Neurofibroma.
    d. Astrocytoma.

97. Which of the following is not true about Bell palsy?
    a. Steroids are the mainstay of treatment.
    b. Permanent neurological deficits may occur.
    c. Bell palsy signals a likely future stroke.
    d. The etiology is unknown.

98. A neonate is diagnosed with herpes encephalitis. What is the most likely cause?
   a. Nosocomial infection.
   b. The infant is immunocompromised.
   c. Iatrogenic cause.
   d. Maternal transmission.

99. A neonate is admitted to the hospital for status epilepticus. After the patient is stabilized, imaging of the brain reveals subdural hematoma, retinal bleeding, and cerebral edema. What is the most likely diagnosis?
   a. Encephalitis.
   b. Shaken baby syndrome.
   c. Meningitis.
   d. Acute disseminating encephalomyelitis.

100. A patient is admitted for possible seizure. Her symptoms do not correspond with findings on electroencephalogram (EEG). Which lab should be ordered to help differentiate between seizure and pseudoseizure?
   a. Prolactin.
   b. Vitamin D.
   c. Sodium.
   d. Erythrocyte sedimentation rate.

101. A child is diagnosed with a traumatic brain injury consistent with abuse. Which of the following is not an appropriate action?
   a. Confront the child's mother about the abuse.
   b. Contact the Division of Youth and Family Services (DYFS) or other local department of child and family services.
   c. Have the patient placed on a 1:1 safety watch while visitors are present.
   d. Consult the case manager and social worker.

102. A patient admitted for stroke has exhibited impulsive behavior. Which of the following is not appropriate to prevent injury?
   a. Soft restraints.
   b. Bed rails.
   c. Sedatives.
   d. 1:1 safety watch.

103. A patient is diagnosed with a hemangioblastoma. The patient inquires what the first-line treatment is for her condition. Which of the following is the correct response?
   a. Chemotherapy.
   b. Radiation.
   c. Palliative care.
   d. Surgical excision.

104. What side effect should medical providers be aware of when administering intravenous phenytoin (Dilantin)?
    a. Blindness.
    b. Malignant hyperthermia.
    c. Hypotension.
    d. Hyperemesis.

105. Which of the following is incorrect regarding Friedreich ataxia?
    a. It is an autosomal dominant disorder.
    b. It increases the risk of scoliosis.
    c. It primarily affects children and young adults.
    d. Most patients require a wheelchair.

106. Which of the following medications should be avoided in a patient with preexisting peripheral neuropathy?
    a. Warfarin (Coumadin).
    b. Phenytoin (Dilantin).
    c. Mannitol (Osmitrol).
    d. Aspirin (Ecotrin).

107. A patient arrives as a possible stroke alert. The patient is lethargic, but able to follow commands. The medical team has sent labs and is bringing the patient for a CT of the head without contrast. What else should be done during a possible stroke workup?
    a. Feed the patient.
    b. Check a C-reactive protein (CRP).
    c. Intubate the patient.
    d. Check blood glucose.

108. An infarction that occurs in the brainstem would affect which of the following functions?
    a. Fine motor function.
    b. Personality.
    c. Memory.
    d. Cardiopulmonary function.

109. A couple arrives in the emergency department following a motor vehicle accident. The wife is awake, alert, and following commands. The husband is lethargic and confused. Which of the following is the most important initial question to ask the wife?
    a. Who was driving?
    b. Is the car totaled?
    c. Does your husband have any underlying medical conditions?
    d. Did your husband lose consciousness?

110. A patient arrives at the emergency department. He opens his eyes to verbal command, is confused, and is not following verbal commands, but has purposeful movements. What is the patient's Glasgow Coma Scale (GCS)?
    a. Eight.
    b. Ten.
    c. Twelve.
    d. Fourteen.

111. A patient with a massive stroke is found to have progressive tachypnea with periods of apnea. What is this phenomenon called?
    a. Cheyne–Stokes breathing.
    b. Wheezing.
    c. Kussmaul breathing.
    d. Stridor.

112. A patient comes to the hospital with facial swelling and ecchymoses 2 days after an assault. The medical practitioner notices ecchymoses over the mastoid process of this patient. What is the most likely underlying injury?
    a. Nasal fracture.
    b. Basilar skull fracture.
    c. Mandibular fracture.
    d. Maxillary fracture.

113. Which medication would most likely be used in a patient in refractory status epilepticus?
    a. Divalproex sodium (Depakote).
    b. Phenytoin (Dilantin).
    c. Levetiracetam (Keppra).
    d. Pentobarbital (Nembutal).

114. A patient experiences a seizure that starts in her arm and continues to her leg on the ipsilateral side. What is this phenomenon called?
    a. Jacksonian march.
    b. Jeffersonian march.
    c. Washington march.
    d. Wilsonian march.

115. Which drug class is generally given in conjunction with antiepileptic drugs?
    a. Benzodiazepines.
    b. Antiplatelet medications.
    c. Narcotics.
    d. Antihistamines.

116. A patient begins to seize while ambulating with the physical therapy team. After lowering the patient to the ground, what is the best way to position the patient to avoid further complications?
    a. Supine.
    b. Prone.
    c. Lateral recumbent.
    d. Dorsal recumbent.

117. A 16-year-old female patient arrives in the emergency department after family members noticed generalized body tremors and eye-rolling. The patient is placed on electroencephalogram (EEG) and admitted for observation. Medical providers note that the patient is awake and talking during these episodes. The EEG is negative for postictal slowing. Which of the following is the most likely diagnosis?
   a. Petit mal seizure.
   b. Complex partial motor seizure.
   c. Grand mal seizure.
   d. Pseudoseizure.

118. Which of the following is not a complication of basilar skull fracture?
   a. Cranial nerve palsy.
   b. Blindness.
   c. Cerebrospinal fluid (CSF) leak.
   d. Deafness.

119. Which of the following is a recommendation given to those with a skull fracture?
   a. Avoid baths.
   b. Do not drive.
   c. Stay on bedrest for 6 weeks.
   d. Avoid blowing your nose.

120. A patient arrives in the ER with a Glasgow Coma Scale (GCS) of 6 after an assault. Which of the following is the most important initial intervention?
   a. Obtain a CT of the head.
   b. Intubate the patient.
   c. Obtain blood work.
   d. Insert a central line.

121. A patient is admitted to the ICU for a large stroke. A woman who states that she is the sister of the patient calls the unit to inquire about the patient's prognosis. Which of the following is the most appropriate action?
   a. Tell the sister that the prognosis is poor.
   b. Politely refuse to give that information.
   c. Give the patient the attending's contact information.
   d. Offer to send the patient's medical records to the woman.

122. An 89-year-old patient presents with aphasia, facial droop, and right-sided hemiparesis that started 4 hours ago. The National Institutes of Health Stroke Scale (NIHSS) is a 32 when evaluated in the emergency department. A CT of the brain shows a large hypodensity in the left middle cerebral artery distribution. Which of the following is the most appropriate action?
   a. Administer tissue plasminogen activator (tPA).
   b. Give aspirin per rectum.
   c. Obtain an MRI of the brain.
   d. Do not give any medication.

123. What is the most common cause of thrombotic stroke?
    a. Hypertension.
    b. Atherosclerosis.
    c. Diabetes mellitus.
    d. Atrial fibrillation.

124. A patient fell off of a ladder and sustained a traumatic brain injury. The patient's Glasgow Coma Scale (GCS) has been a 5 for the past week. The patient's spouse inquires about the best course of action. What is the most appropriate response?
    a. The patient should undergo brain death protocol.
    b. The patient should be on comfort measures only (CMO).
    c. The patient would benefit from a brain injury rehabilitation program.
    d. The patient may benefit from a trial of ventilation weaning.

125. A young man in the clinic for bronchitis makes intermittent barking noises while having a conversation with a medical provider. His exam is otherwise normal. What is the most likely diagnosis?
    a. Simple motor seizure.
    b. Tardive dyskinesia.
    c. Tourette syndrome.
    d. Complex motor seizure.

126. Which of the following is medication used to treat restless leg syndrome (RLS)?
    a. Ropinirole (Requip).
    b. Labetalol (Trandate).
    c. Haloperidol (Haldol).
    d. Esmolol (Brevibloc).

127. A patient with untreated sleep apnea is at risk for which of the following?
    a. Diffuse axonal injury (DAI).
    b. Subarachnoid hemorrhage (SAH).
    c. Stroke.
    d. Abscess.

128. Which of the following is not an appropriate intervention for a patient with a history of chemical dependency who has recently had a stroke?
    a. Provide a rolling walker to help restore mobility.
    b. Refer to a physical therapist.
    c. Recommend lifestyle changes.
    d. Offer to be the patient's sponsor.

129. A patient comes to the ER complaining of headache, nausea, vomiting, and tremors. There is a known history of alcohol abuse, but the patient denies drinking for the past 2 days. Which of the following is a common complication of this patient's condition?
    a. Seizure.
    b. Stroke.
    c. Intracerebral hemorrhage.
    d. Abscess.

130. A 35-year-old man who recently emigrated from Guatemala presents with seizure. He has no history of seizure. Prior to moving to the United States he raised animals, primarily pigs, on his farm. MRI of the brain reveals multiple ring-enhancing cystic lesions. Which of the following is a common complication of this patient's condition?
    a. Bony metastases.
    b. Stroke.
    c. Intracerebral hemorrhage.
    d. Hydrocephalus.

131. Which of the following is not a relative contraindication for tissue plasminogen activator (tPA)?
    a. Recent lumbar puncture.
    b. Serum glucose < 50 mg/dL.
    c. History of gastrointestinal hemorrhage 2 weeks ago.
    d. Pregnancy.

132. Which of the following statements regarding tissue plasminogen activator (tPA) is not correct?
    a. It can be used up to 4.5 hours after stroke symptom onset.
    b. It can be used in pregnant women.
    c. It increases the risk of hemorrhagic stroke.
    d. It can be used in patients 16 years of age and older.

133. What is the most common cause for an embolic stroke?
    a. Atherosclerosis.
    b. Hypertension.
    c. Atrial fibrillation.
    d. Diabetes mellitus.

134. Which of the following is a highly malignant central nervous system neoplasm in infants/children?
    a. Rhabdoid tumor.
    b. Meningioma.
    c. Acoustic neuroma.
    d. Ependymoma.

135. Which of the following is the most common type of primary bone malignancy?
    a. Osteochondroma.
    b. Osteosarcoma.
    c. Malignant giant cell tumor.
    d. Chordoma.

136. Which of the following is not a treatment used for multiple sclerosis?
    a. Baclofen (Lioresal).
    b. Beta interferons.
    c. Prednisone (Deltasone).
    d. Haloperidol (Haldol).

137. What is the most common type of cancer to metastasize to the bone?
    a. Ovarian.
    b. Brain.
    c. Breast.
    d. Colorectal.

138. A patient has a subdural hematoma following a fall 2 weeks ago. Which of the following is the correct diagnosis?
    a. Acute subdural.
    b. Acute on chronic subdural.
    c. Subacute subdural.
    d. Chronic subdural.

139. A patient receiving tissue plasminogen activator (tPA) begins to seize. The vital signs remain stable throughout the seizure. Which of the following is the initial step in treatment?
    a. Discontinue the tPA.
    b. Place the patient on an electroencephalogram (EEG).
    c. Administer an anticonvulsant drug.
    d. Intubate the patient.

140. Which of the following is false regarding rhabdoid tumors?
    a. Macrocephaly is a common presenting symptom.
    b. Radiation therapy is the treatment of choice.
    c. Prognosis is poor.
    d. Common location is in the cerebral hemisphere.

141. Which of the following is not a predisposing factor for development of a cerebral aneurysm?
    a. Tobacco abuse.
    b. Asian ancestry.
    c. Hypertension.
    d. Females.

142. Optic neuritis is most closely associated with which of the following conditions?
    a. Amyotrophic lateral sclerosis.
    b. Posterior reversible encephalopathy syndrome.
    c. Myasthenia gravis.
    d. Multiple sclerosis.

143. A patient arrives in the ER with left facial droop and left arm paresthesia. The symptoms resolved prior to arrival at the hospital. The NIHSS is zero in the ER. Which of the following is not an appropriate treatment?
    a. Check serum glucose.
    b. Obtain a CT of the head.
    c. Discharge the patient home.
    d. Obtain a urine drug screen.

144. What is a major complication of vasospasm in an aneurysmal subarachnoid hemorrhage (SAH) patient?
    a. Abscess.
    b. Optic neuritis.
    c. Stroke.
    d. Hearing loss.

145. Which of the following is true about acoustic neuromas?
    a. A common presenting symptom is balance difficulty.
    b. It is a malignant tumor.
    c. It is a common condition.
    d. Tobacco abuse is a risk factor.

146. A patient with a traumatic brain injury is being examined by the medical team. On physical exam, the person is stiff with bent arms, clenched fists, and legs held out straight. The arms are bent in toward the body and the wrists and fingers are bent and held on the chest. Which of the following would best describe the patient's exam?
    a. Contracted.
    b. Decorticate posturing.
    c. Withdrawing.
    d. Decerebrate posturing.

147. Regular oral hygiene is an essential intervention for the client who has had a stroke. Which of the following nursing measures is inappropriate when providing oral hygiene?
    a. Have the patient lie supine while rinsing their mouth.
    b. Keep portable suction equipment at the bedside.
    c. Explain each step of personal hygiene in slow clear voice.
    d. Clean the patient's mouth with a toothbrush.

148. A patient arrives in the ER with left-sided paresthesia and dysarthria 1 hour prior to arrival. The NIHSS was 10 prior to the patient going for CT of the head. The NIHSS was 1 after the patient returned from CT scan. Which of the following is the most appropriate action?
    a. Give tissue plasminogen activator (tPA).
    b. Give warfarin.
    c. Give aspirin.
    d. Do not give medication.

149. A patient arrives in the hospital with a possible stroke. Which of the following questions is the most important initial question?
    a. Do you have a power of attorney?
    b. Do you have any allergies?
    c. What is the time of symptom onset?
    d. Have you ever had these symptoms before?

150. A patient has just been given tissue plasminogen activator (tPA). Which of the following vital signs is the most crucial to monitor?
    a. Respiratory rate.
    b. Cerebral perfusion pressure (CPP).
    c. Pulse oximetry.
    d. Mean arterial pressure (MAP).

151. Which of the following is the most important physical assessment to monitor in someone who has just received tissue plasminogen activator (tPA)?
    a. Corneal reflexes.
    b. Motor strength.
    c. Cardiac exam.
    d. Rectal exam.

152. A patient has a stroke. During the hospital stay, he is also diagnosed with new-onset atrial fibrillation. Which of the following drugs will most likely be prescribed for the patient?
    a. Warfarin (Coumadin).
    b. Amlodipine (Norvasc).
    c. Losartan (Cozaar).
    d. Furosemide (Lasix).

153. Which of the following patients is at the highest risk for stroke?
    a. 50-year-old African American man with cocaine abuse.
    b. 65-year-old Caucasian woman with hypertension.
    c. 70-year-old Asian man with no past medical history.
    d. 55-year-old African American woman with chronic anemia.

154. The medical team is evaluating a patient who was involved in a motor collision. The team notices involuntary extension of the arms and legs with the toes pointed downward. Which of the following best describes the exam findings?
    a. Contracted.
    b. Decorticate posturing.
    c. Withdrawing.
    d. Decerebrate posturing.

155. A patient comes to the ER with right hemiparesis that developed 3.5 hours ago. The blood pressure is 170/90 mm Hg, the heart rate is 120 bpm, and the serum glucose is 550 mg/dL. Which of the following is a contraindication to administration of thrombolytics?
    a. Symptom onset.
    b. Blood pressure.
    c. Heart rate.
    d. Serum glucose.

156. A patient with left hemiparesis due to a recent stroke is noted to have poor oral intake. Which of the following is the not an appropriate intervention?
    a. Encourage the patient to feed himself.
    b. Have an orderly assist with feedings.
    c. Obtain a speech pathology consult for dysphagia evaluation.
    d. Order a calorie count.

157. A health care provider performs a neurological exam on a suspected stroke patient. The patient is having difficulty with the finger to nose test. What is this physical examination finding called?
    a. Tardive dyskinesia.
    b. Dysmetria.
    c. Ataxia.
    d. Dysarthria.

158. A patient admitted with a significant traumatic brain injury is about to be discharged and the medical team is teaching the patient's husband about safety precautions. Which of the following actions shows that he understands instructions?
    a. Leaving the bed rails down.
    b. Inspecting the entire body for skin breakdown.
    c. Having the patient feed herself.
    d. Leaving the wheelchair brakes unlocked.

159. A patient is admitted for stroke. During his neurologic assessment, the nurse notices that that patient waddles with his legs wide apart. What type of gait disturbance is this called?
    a. Helicopod.
    b. Ataxic.
    c. Dystrophic.
    d. Parkinsonian.

160. A patient is admitted to the hospital for significant traumatic brain injury. Which of the following maneuvers is appropriate to assess corneal reflexes?
    a. Have the patient follow a stimulus with their eyes.
    b. Shine a light into the patient's eyes.
    c. Drop saline into the patient's eyes.
    d. Apply sternomastoid pressure.

161. A 68-year-old African American woman with a history of obesity and diabetes mellitus presents to the ER with left facial droop. Which of the following is not a risk factor for stroke?
    a. Race.
    b. Sex.
    c. Diabetes mellitus.
    d. Obesity.

162. A patient with a suspected stroke is about to get an MRI of the brain. The patient states that she is claustrophobic. Which of the following interventions is not appropriate prior to obtaining the MRI?
    a. Check history to ensure the patient does not have any metallic devices.
    b. Reassure the patient.
    c. Give the patient a benzodiazepine.
    d. Feed the patient.

163. A patient with a traumatic brain injury is noted to have impulsive behavior. Which of the following is the most appropriate initial intervention?
    a. Psychiatry consult.
    b. 1:1 safety watch.
    c. Restraints.
    d. Redirection of behavior.

164. For a patient with elevated intracranial pressure (ICP), the primary goal is which of the following?
    a. Place the patient in a hypothermic coma.
    b. Lower the patient's blood pressure.
    c. Increase the patient's oxygenation levels.
    d. Eliminate carbon dioxide.

165. A patient with a suspected stroke is ordered to undergo an MRI of the brain. The patient has a history of cataract surgery, permanent pacemaker, cholecystectomy, and a vasectomy. Which of the following prohibits the patient from getting an MRI?
    a. Cataract surgery.
    b. Permanent pacemaker.
    c. Cholecystectomy.
    d. Vasectomy.

# Answers and Explanations

1. D: Maintaining the airway is the most important factor in any situation. Although all postictal patients do not need to be intubated, if the patient is significantly lethargic, short-term respiratory support may be needed until neurological status returns to baseline. An electrocardiogram can be performed once the patient has stabilized. If the patient has sufficient peripheral access, a central line is not warranted. If the patient does not have sufficient access and the medical team is unable to place a peripheral line, an interosseous line can be placed in the interim. Depending on the suspected etiology of the seizure, a lumbar puncture may not be needed.

2. C: A petite mal or absence seizure is characterized by persistent staring episodes. These types of seizures are normally seen in children. A partial seizure only affects one area of the body. A patient does not lose consciousness during these types of seizures. Pseudoseizures are characterized by seizure-like activity but are nonepileptic in etiology. They are generally caused by extreme stress or a desire for attention.

3. B: Previous guidelines recommend administration of tissue plasminogen activator (tPA) for acute ischemic stroke within 3 hours of stroke symptom onset. Recent guidelines have shown that the window can extended up to 4.5 hours. The patient's age, history of recent abdominal surgery, and blood pressure are relative contraindications. Intracranial hemorrhage, recent head trauma in the last 3 months, active internal bleeding, uncontrolled blood pressure (more than 185/100 mm Hg), abnormal clotting factors due to malignancy or anticoagulation (INR more than 1.7, platelet count less than 100,000/mm$^3$), glucose less than 50 mg/dL or more than 400 mg/dL, and seizure at stroke onset are other absolute contraindications to tPA.

4. A: Dark green, leafy vegetables are excellent sources of vitamin K, which enables the blood to form clots. It acts against warfarin. Patients on warfain are advised to eat green, leafy vegetables in moderation and to keep the intake consistent. Recent research has shown that consistent low intake of vitamin K may prevent fluctuations in international normalized ratio (INR).

5. B: Coagulation panel and platelet count are important labs to check prior to any invasive procedure. If there are abnormalities in the lab, they should be addressed or corrected prior to the procedure to help prevent complications. The patient should lie on their side in the fetal position or be sitting hunched for optimal positioning. Having central access is not needed as long as the patient has sufficient peripheral access. Making sure that the patient has used the bathroom is important, but not the most important nursing procedure.

6. A: Cushing triad is defined as irregular respirations, bradycardia, and hypertension; it is a physiologic nervous system response to persistent increased intracranial pressure (ICP). Normal ICPs measure < 20 mm Hg. It is a sign of impending herniation. Other signs and symptoms may include altered mental status, fixed or unequal pupils, nausea, vomiting, headache, and seizure.

7. A: Clinicians should advise their patients to eat several small meals per day to prevent aspiration. Myasthenia gravis is a chronic autoimmune neuromuscular disease that affects the body's voluntary musculature. Antibodies attack normal acetylcholine receptors. The signature issue is fluctuating muscle weakness. Signs and symptoms may include facial weakness causing droop or ptosis, dysphagia, extremity weakness, ataxia, impaired speech, visual difficulties, and shortness of breath. Treatments for myasthenia gravis include immunosuppressive medications, plasmapheresis, and cholinesterase inhibitors.

8. C: An MRI scan is the diagnostic test that will give definitive diagnosis for Chiari malformation. Other imaging tests such as CT scan, ultrasound, and PET scan are not sensitive enough to detect this abnormality. In Chiari malformations, the lower part of the cerebellum herniates through the base of the skull. There are three types of Chiari malformation (I, II, and III). The simplest and most common is Chiari I. Most Chiari I birth defects are present at birth, though symptoms may not become apparent for some time. Chiari II and III are more severe. Birth defects that are associated with other brain and spinal cord birth defects, such as spina bifida, are apparent at birth.

9. A: Headaches following a lumbar puncture are the most common complication of the procedure. Postlumbar puncture headache is caused by leakage of cerebrospinal fluid from the dura, exacerbated in an upright position and improved in the supine position. Clinicians should recommend that the patient lie flat for several hours following the procedure to help minimize complications.

10. D: Calling the attending/resident/physician's assistant on call is appropriate because the patient's ICP is high and the drain is not working. There may be a clot in the drain, which may or may not need to be flushed (this should not be done by the nurse). There are other reasons why a drain may not be working and it is up to the attending to decide what the next step should be. A normal ICP should be between 0 and 20. A sustained ICP of 30 may cause permanent brain injury; monitoring it without calling an attending is inappropriate.

11. C: Normal pressure hydrocephalus (NPH) is a neurological abnormality of unknown etiology that results in abnormal CSF on the brain. The clinical triad is dementia, ataxia, and urinary incontinence. Diagnostic tests include CT scan or MRI of the brain and lumbar puncture. If a lumbar puncture results in improvement or resolution of symptoms, then the patient may likely need a ventriculoperitoneal shunt (VPS). A Tinetti assessment is usually performed by physical therapists and measures the stability and mobility of a patient. Patients with encephalitis or meningitis do not have symptoms that improve following a lumbar puncture and their symptoms are not measured by a Tinetti assessment. Posterior reversible encephalopathy syndrome (PRES) is a neurological disorder that resolves once the underlying cause is treated (i.e. hypertension).

12. B: The limbic system is responsible for emotions and memory. The occipital cortex is primarily responsible for vision. The centers for speech are primarily located in the temporal lobes. The frontal lobes are primarily responsible for decision-making, and impulse control is located in the frontal cortex.

13. A: Aspirin and ticagrelor are antiplatelet medications that can increase the risk of excessive bleeding. They prevent cells from clotting together too readily to help prevent thromboembolic events. Patients should be advised that if they notice chronic excessive bleeding to notify a clinician immediately.

14. A: Hypertonic fluids would be used to decrease intracranial pressure (ICP). Hypertonic fluid such as 3% NaCl is used for severe hyponatremia (serum Na less than 125 mEq/L) and patients with cerebral edema. Persistent elevated ICP can cause global brain ischemia and eventual brain death. The brain is 80% water, so agents such as hypertonic saline and osmotic diuretics draw cerebrospinal fluid out of the cranium and fluid out of the injured brain, reducing pressure and further injury. Agitation and pain can contribute to elevated ICP so analgesics and sedatives are commonly used. Hyperventilation may also be used to decrease ICP. Hyperventilation decreases $PaCO_2$, which can induce constriction of cerebral arteries, which decreases ICP by reducing blood flow volume.

15. A: Creutzfeldt–Jakob disease is a rare progressive neurological disorder transmitted primarily by ingesting contaminated meat. Some cases are genetic. The initial presentation of symptoms may include confusion, agitation, and hallucinations. As the disease progresses, the patient develops seizures, ataxia, involuntary jerking movements, and dysphagia. They become unable to care for themselves, requiring a feeding tube and sometimes mechanical ventilation.

16. B: A central stimulus is an area on the body where the brain is involved in the response to the pain. Examples of central stimuli include the face and chest. A peripheral stimulus is an area of the body where the brain is not involved in the response to pain. It can be also induced as a result of reflex. Examples of peripheral stimuli include the fingers, toes, elbows, and knees.

17. D: Face mask, gown, and gloves are needed to help prevent the spread of meningitis. Handwashing is the most important universal precaution, but it was not offered as an option in this scenario. Meningitis is spread through secretions such as saliva and mucus. A face mask should be worn at all times when treating someone with suspected or confirmed meningitis. Gloves and a gown are additional precautions in case a person touches their clothing or face after handling a patient with meningitis.

18. A: A grand mal seizure or a generalized tonic-clonic seizure is usually preceded by an aura, followed by eye -rolling, drooling, incontinence, and uncontrolled tremors, followed by a postictal period. A petit mal seizure is another term for absence seizure. This type of seizure is typically seen in children and involves blank staring episodes and loss of consciousness. A simple partial seizure involves an extremity without loss of consciousness or postictal period.

19. C: The patient has meningitis, which can usually be confirmed by lumbar puncture. The Brudzinski sign is characterized by severe neck stiffness causing the patient's hips and knees to flex when the neck is flexed. This is due to the irritation of the meninges. Blood cultures and a CAT scan of the chest, abdomen, and pelvis have no diagnostic value in evaluating meningitis. The ESR may be elevated, but it is a nonspecific marker of inflammation.

20. B: Glioblastoma multiforme (GBM) is the most common primary brain tumor in American adults. The symptoms are nonspecific. They may include headache, nausea, vomiting, ataxia, and dizziness. The etiology is unknown. Risk factors include advanced age, male, and certain neurologic conditions such as neurofibromatosis. GBMs can be diagnosed with MRI, but biopsy provides definitive diagnosis. Treatment depends on tumor grade.

21. C: Meningiomas are usually benign masses. In this case, the meningioma was an incidental finding during a trauma workup. If a meningioma is large enough to cause symptoms, a craniotomy and debulking may be performed. In this case, repeat imaging is the best initial course of action.

22. C: The frontal cortex is primarily responsible for decision-making, problem solving, control of purposeful behaviors, and voluntary movements. The pineal gland regulates the daily and seasonal circadian rhythms, the sleep-wake patterns that determine hormone levels, stress levels, and physical performance. The hypothalamus has many important physiologic functions such as formation of memories, temperature regulation, thirst, mood, and the release of other hormones within the body. The basal ganglia help coordinate fine motor movements.

23. A: Ethosuximide (Zarontin) is the first-line therapy for treating absence or petit mal seizures. This type of seizure is typically seen in children and involves blank staring episodes and loss of

consciousness. Phenytoin is used to treat and prevent tonic-clonic seizures and status epilepticus. Levetiracetam is used to prevent tonic-clonic and simple partial seizures. Lacosamide is used to treat simple partial seizures.

24. A: An epidural hematoma is the accumulation of blood between the dura mater and the skull as a result of severe blunt force trauma. It appears as a convex hypodensity on imaging of the brain. It usually requires surgical evacuation. A subarachnoid hemorrhage is accumulation of blood in the arachnoid space between the skull and the pia mater. It appears as a lacy reticular pattern. This may be due to trauma or aneurysmal rupture. Treatment depends on etiology. A subdural hematoma is the accumulation of blood between the dura mater and the surface of the brain. It may occur due to blunt force trauma or may occur spontaneously, especially in those on long-term anticoagulation therapy. It appears as a concave hypodensity on brain imaging. Treatment generally involves surgical evacuation. Hemorrhagic contusions are superficial contusions on the brain's surface due to trauma. They do not require surgery.

25. D: Patients only need to wear craniectomy helmets when out of bed to protect their skull in case of a fall. The portion of their brain by the surgical site no longer has skull to protect it in the event of injury.

26. D: Mannitol is an osmotic diuretic and would be used to help decrease ICP. Persistent elevated ICP can cause global brain ischemia and eventual brain death. The brain is 80% water, so agents such as hypertonic saline and osmotic diuretics draw cerebrospinal fluid out of the cranium and fluid out of the injured brain, reducing pressure and further injury.

27. C: Anticoagulation and antiplatelet medications should be held for 24 hours following tPA administration (also known as the tPA window) until a follow-up CT scan is negative for hemorrhage. No invasive lines such a central lines or nasogastric tubes should be placed since the patient is at increased risk of bleeding. Once the 24-hour window has passed, a nasogastric tube may be placed if the patient continues to fail swallow evaluations.

28. C: Tube feeds would be the most appropriate recommendation. These may be given through a nasogastric tube until a patient passes a swallow evaluation or until a feeding tube may be placed. If the patient's gut is working, total parental nutrition should be avoided to avoid gut atrophy.

29. B: A subdural hematoma is the accumulation of blood between the dura mater and the surface of the brain. It may occur due to blunt force trauma or spontaneously, especially in those on long-term anticoagulation therapy. It appears as a concave hypodensity on brain imaging. Treatment generally involves surgical evacuation. Hemorrhagic contusions are superficial contusions on the brain's surface due to trauma. They do not require surgery. An epidural hematoma is the accumulation of blood between the dura mater and the skull as a result of severe blunt force trauma. It appears as a convex hypodensity on imaging of the brain. It usually requires surgical evacuation. Diffuse axonal injury is the shearing of tiny blood vessels in the brain due to blunt trauma. It appears on MRI and punctate diffuse microhemorrhages. Treatment involves conservative management.

30. A: Triple-H therapy (hypervolemia, hemodilution, and hypertension) aims to increase cerebral perfusion in aneurysmal subarachnoid hemorrhage and helps prevent vasospasm.

31. A: Lordosis is an abnormality of the spine that causes chronic back pain. It is characterized by the excessive straightening of the cervical and/or thoracic spine and exaggerated inward curvature

of the lumbar spine. Spondylolisthesis is a condition in which the vertebrae in the lower back slip forward. Kyphosis is the exaggerated outward curvature of the thoracic spine, causing a hunchback appearance. Scoliosis is the abnormal sideways curvature of the spine, giving it an 'S' shaped appearance on imaging.

32. C: Trigeminal neuralgia is an impingement of the trigeminal nerve or facial nerve causing intermittent severe sharp facial pain with stimulation. This pain may be exacerbated by something as simple as chewing gum, putting on makeup, eating a crunchy snack, or drinking a cold beverage.

33. D: Increasing the respiratory rate, causing a decrease in carbon dioxide is the most appropriate intervention for high ICP. A normal mean arterial pressure (MAP) ranges between 60 and 100 mm Hg. A normal ICP ranges between 0 and 20 mm Hg. Cerebral perfusion pressure (CPP) is the net pressure driving blood flow to the brain. The brain needs a minimum of 60 mm Hg before neuronal cell death starts to occur. CPP is measured by ICP from the MAP. In this scenario, the patient's CPP is 56. Carbon dioxide dilates the cerebral blood vessels, increasing the volume of blood in the brain. Hyperventilation decreases $CO_2$, which will help decrease the ICP. Decreasing the $FiO_2$ will cause further brain damage since the patient already has high ICP. A high PEEP can increase ICP by impeding cerebral blood flow.

34. B: Low-sodium diets are recommended for those with Meniere disease. The etiology is unknown, but it is believed that abnormal fluid buildup in the inner ear causes Meniere disease. Signs and symptoms may include vertigo, tinnitus, and progressive hearing loss. It is generally advised that patients with this condition maintain a low-sodium diet to help lower the fluid level and pressure in the inner ear.

35. B: Arteriovenous malformations (AVMs) are mostly idiopathic. People are born with this condition and may be asymptomatic their entire lives. However, if an AVM becomes large enough or ruptures, it may cause significant neurological deficits, coma, and death. An AVM is an abnormal growth of arteries that shunt directly into a vein. The high pressure system of the arterial blood flow causes the low pressure vein to expand and possibly rupture.

36. B: Scheuermann disease or Scheuermann kyphosis is caused by the uneven growth of the vertebra, which causes kyphosis in children. Most deformities are corrected with braces, but in severe cases surgical intervention is warranted. Pott disease, or tuberculous spondylitis, is where tuberculosis affects the spine, causing chronic arthritis and pathologic fractures. Amyotrophic lateral sclerosis (ALS), also known as Lou Gehrig's disease, is a progressive neurodegenerative disorder that causes muscle weakness, paralysis, dysphagia, and respiratory insufficiency. Neurofibromatosis is an autosomal dominant condition in which tumors develop in the central nervous system.

37. D: Obtaining a CBC is the most important lab to obtain out of the choices given. The surgeon needs to know the hemoglobin and hematocrit as well as the platelet count prior to the procedure. An ESR would provide little value since it is a nonspecific marker of inflammation. Liver function tests would provide little value since the patient has no history of medical problems and these would likely be normal. A BMP is probably the second most important lab. Since the patient is young and has no past medical history, his BUN and creatinine, as well as electrolytes, are likely normal.

38. D: A subdural hematoma is the accumulation of blood between the dura mater and the surface of the brain. It may occur due to blunt force trauma or spontaneously. It appears as a concave

hypodensity on brain imaging. Subacute bleeds occur 2 to 4 weeks following an incident. Chronic bleeds appear after 4 weeks following an incident. An epidural hematoma is the accumulation of blood between the dura mater and the skull as a result of severe blunt force trauma. It appears as a convex hypodensity on imaging of the brain.

39. D: Repeat imaging in the next 6 to 12 months would be the most appropriate intervention for a tiny unruptured aneurysm. Aneurysms larger than 5 to 6 mm require surgical repair. Imaging of the chest and abdomen would provide no value.

40. A: A patient who has lost their brainstem reflexes would be appropriate for brain death protocol. This involves imaging with a radioactive isotope to illustrate whether or not there is blood flow to the brain. This test in conjunction with an apnea test will prove that the patient is brain dead. Prior to initiating brain death protocol, a clinician must be able to document the cause of the vegetative state. In this case, it was severe trauma. The patient's body temperature must be normal or near normal, the patient cannot be on paralytic or sedative medications, and there should be no acid-base or endocrine disorders.

41. C: A palliative care consult is the most reasonable intervention in this scenario. The patient is an elderly patient with an incurable diagnosis and is refusing intervention that will prolong life. Since this patient is neurologically intact, they have the right to make their own decisions regarding their health care. The palliative care team may help the spouse come to terms with the patient's diagnosis and explain hospice care.

42. B: Ependymomas form from ependymal cells that line the ventricles. These cells are responsible for making cerebrospinal fluid. In children, these tumors are generally intracranial, and in adults they generally form in the spine. Acoustic neuromas, also known as vestibular schwannomas, grow around the eighth cranial nerve and present with hearing changes and balance difficulties. Brainstem gliomas are found at the base of the brain and may cause speech, vision, or coordination abnormalities.

43. C: Referral to an audiologist is recommended for those with neurofibromatosis. Neurofibromatosis occurs due to a genetic defect that causes tumors to arise from nerve cells. Complications that may occur from this disorder include deafness, hypertension, seizures, hydrocephalus, scoliosis, pathologic fractures, kyphosis, and vision problems.

44. A: Amyotrophic lateral sclerosis (ALS) is a progressive neurodegenerative disorder that presents with muscle atrophy, weakness, dysphagia, and respiratory insufficiency, and progresses to the patient being immobile and on a ventilator. There is no way to effectively halt or treat the progression of this disease. The goal of care is to keep the patient comfortable and mobile for as long as possible.

45. D: The patient has a history of facial fractures that predispose to infection. The bacteria that normally reside in the sinuses now have a pathway to the brain. Brain abscesses as well as certain masses such as meningiomas can appear as ring-enhancing masses on imaging. However, the patient's history of trauma and current presentation with fever are more consistent with an infectious etiology.

46. C: Plasmapheresis is one of the treatment modalities used for Guillain-Barré syndrome. It is an autoimmune disease that affects the nerves that can lead to weakness and paralysis. It is usually preceded by an illness such as influenza. Pyridostigmine is used to treat myasthenia gravis. Aspirin

and penicillin can be used to treat multiple conditions, but are not used in the treatment of Guillain-Barré syndrome.

47. C: Frontal headaches are generally not associated with vertebral artery dissection. The vertebral arteries are located in the back of the neck, which forms the basilar artery. They are part of the posterior circulation of the brain. Patients with a vertebral artery dissection can present with TIA symptoms or posterior stroke. They may present with visual changes since the vision centers are located in the visual cortex. Other symptoms may include neck pain or posterior headache.

48. B: The patient has failed medical therapy and needs surgical intervention. The patient has had several TIAs and has moderate stenosis of his right internal carotid artery; he is at very high risk for future stroke. Ticagrelor and clopidogrel are in the same drug category. They are used as alternatives to one another, but are never used together. Administration of tPA is not warranted since the patient's symptoms resolved. TPA is never given for TIAs. If the patient refused to undergo surgery or was not a surgical candidate, changing the clopidogrel to warfarin may be an option.

49. C: Hydrocephalus is a concern with intraventricular hemorrhage (IVH) since it is the area where cerebrospinal fluid (CSF) is produced. This results in obstructive hydrocephalus. Abscesses would be incredibly uncommon unless the patient was immunocompromised. Blindness is generally caused by pathology in the posterior circulation/structures. Seizures are not common in deep subcortical pathology.

50. A: Chronic hypertension is the most common cause of lacunar infarcts. Lacunar stroke is a type of ischemic stroke that occurs when blood flow to one of the small arterial vessels deep within the brain becomes blocked.

51. C: The patient does not need to be on bed rest. Reasonable physical activity as tolerated is encouraged in both in-patient and out-patient settings for stroke patients to help them improve their range of motion, ambulation, and strength. Recommending bed rest will only exacerbate their residual deficits caused by the stroke and increase the risk for deep vein thromboses, decubitus ulcers, and atelectasis.

52. D: Esomeprazole and clopidogrel should not be taken together since esomeprazole can blunt the effect of clopidogrel. Esomeprazole blocks an enzyme in the body that turns clopidogrel into its active form. For patients who have gastroesophageal reflux disease and need to also take clopidogrel, famotidine and pantoprazole are good alternatives that do not affect clopidogrel.

53. D: Iceberg lettuce is very low in vitamin K. Dark green, leafy vegetables such as chard, spinach, kale, brussel sprouts, and collard greens contain high levels of vitamin K and should be eaten in limited quantities. Natural supplements such as ginger and cranberries can also prolong bleeding time and can affect warfarin. Alcohol should be avoided because it can increase the risk of falls, which is particularly problematic for those taking blood thinners. Alcohol can also prolong bleeding time and can affect warfarin.

54. D: The prolonged use on anticonvulsants in children with febrile seizures is not recommended. In recurrent cases, a doctor may recommend that a child take a benzodiazepine along with ibuprofen or acetaminophen when they begin developing a fever. Febrile seizures are do not fall under the category of epilepsy because epilepsy is defined as the presence of recurrent seizures without a particular cause or trigger. Febrile seizures are relatively common in infants and toddlers.

They are generally rare in children younger than 2 or 3 months and children who are older than 4 years of age. The older a child is when they have their first febrile seizure, the decreased likelihood that they will have more in the future. Febrile seizures generally do not have any sequelae; the biggest risk with febrile seizures is aspiration.

55. A: D5W (dextrose 5% in water) contains 5 percent dextrose in water, which is a hypotonic solution. It draws water out of the circulation and into the cells. This is a problem in patients with intracerebral hemorrhages, vasogenic edema, and/or patients with high intracranial pressure because this can exacerbate their condition. D5W should never be ordered in these patients. The other options are either isotonic solutions (normal saline and lactated Ringer's) or hypertonic solutions (3% NaCl), which are acceptable to use in brain injury patients.

56. B: The patient is in a persistent vegetative state due to diffuse axonal injury (DAI), which is caused by shearing of the small blood vessels in the brain following an assault or high speed collision. CT scans may miss the findings associated with DAI. MRIs are the test of choice since they are more sensitive. Findings of DAI are similar to those with MS; however, due to the history of trauma, DAI is the most likely diagnosis. Subdural hematomas (SDHs) and subarachnoid hemorrhages (SAHs) are easily picked up on CT scan. SDHs appear as a concave hypodensity and SAHs appear as a lacy reticular pattern on CT.

57. A: Brown-Sequard syndrome is caused by damage to one-half of the spinal cord, resulting in paralysis and loss of proprioception on the ipsilateral side of the injury, and loss of pain and temperature sensation on the contralateral side of the injury. As an incomplete spinal cord syndrome, the neurological damage may range from mild to significant.

58. C: All of the choices given may cause spondylolisthesis, but trauma is the least common cause. Spondylolisthesis is the forward displacement of a vertebra. Isthmic spondylolisthesis is the most common form. A slip of the intravertebral joint may occur as early as childhood and symptoms may not appear until later in life. It is usually treated with conservative management, although surgical fusion may be warranted if symptoms are significant and refractory to conservative measures.

59. A: A C2 fracture will cause significant deficits, requiring an indwelling catheter for incontinence, a tracheostomy for respiratory insufficiency, a PEG tube for feeding, and complete assistance with activities of daily living, such as eating, dressing, bathing, and getting in or out of bed. A patient with a C7 fracture may be able to breathe and speak normally. Most people can straighten their arm and have normal movement of their shoulders. They may be able to feed themselves with some assistance. Those with thoracic fractures may paraplegic, but can manage most activities of daily life independently and will likely not need a feeding tube.

60. B: The patient most likely has a temporal bone fracture that is causing his cerebrospinal fluid (CSF) leak. The temporal bones enclose many vital structures, including the cochlear and vestibular end organs. If damaged, an abnormal passage is created, allowing CSF to drain into the ear. The halo sign or bull's eye sign is a classic image seen with CSF leaks. Different components of a fluid will separate as it travels through a material, creating a halo or a bull's eye appearance.

61. D: Although all of these factors increase the risk of having a stroke, atrial fibrillation (AF) can increase the risk of stroke 4 times than a person who does not have AF. The irregular contractions of the heart can produce tiny clots that may cause an embolic stroke. Those with AF need to be closely monitored to ensure that they are maximized on medical therapy.

62. C: Hemangioblastomas are benign tumors that occur in the blood vessels in the central nervous system. If they are large or cause symptoms, they may be removed via surgical excision or through Gamma Knife technology. Since the hemangioma was discovered as an incidental finding, serial imaging would be the most appropriate course of management.

63. A: Renal cell carcinoma, breast cancer, and lung cancer are the most likely malignancies to spread to the brain. Lymphomas, genitourinary cancers, colorectal cancer, and pancreatic cancer are significantly less likely to spread to the brain.

64. B: C7 is most likely affected. A patient with a C7 fracture may be able to breathe and speak normally. Most people can straighten their arm and have normal movement of their shoulders. They may be able to feed themselves with some assistance and can operate a motorized wheelchair. A C2 fracture will cause significant deficits, requiring an indwelling catheter for incontinence, a tracheostomy for respiratory insufficiency, a PEG tube for feeding, and complete assistance with activities of daily living, such as eating, dressing, bathing, and getting in or out of bed. Those with thoracic fractures may be paraplegic, but can manage most activities of daily life independently. They can generally operate a manual wheelchair and have normal function of their arms and hands.

65. A: This child most likely has acute disseminated encephalomyelitis (ADEM). ADEM is an immune-mediated inflammatory demyelinating condition that typically resolves with aggressive steroid administration. If treated quickly and appropriately, there are generally no sequelae. ADEM is usually seen following a viral infection or administration of a vaccine. Chronic inflammatory demyelinating polyneuropathy (CIDP) is the chronic form of Guillain-Barré syndrome. Myasthenia gravis is an autoimmune condition characterized by waxing and waning voluntary muscle weakness. ALS is a progressive neurodegenerative disease seen in middle-aged or older adults; it rarely affects children.

66. A: A simple partial seizure involves one or both extremities on a unilateral distribution without loss of consciousness or postictal period. A complex partial seizure also seizure involves one or both extremities on a unilateral distribution. In contrast to a simple partial seizure, it includes preceding symptoms such as lip smacking or eye-rolling and loss of consciousness followed by a postictal period. A petit mal seizure is another term for absence seizure. This type of seizure is typically seen in children, involving blank staring episodes and loss of consciousness. These episodes can occur up to several times a day whereas complex partial seizures usually occur a few times a week. A grand mal seizure or a generalized tonic-clonic seizure is usually preceded by an aura, followed by eye-rolling, drooling, incontinence, and uncontrolled tremors, followed by a postictal period.

67. C: MRI of the brain without gadolinium is the most diagnostic radiologic tool. Characteristic radiographic findings include bilateral regions of subcortical vasogenic edema that resolve within days or weeks on repeat imaging. Patients frequently present with headache, nausea, vomiting, altered mental status, seizures, stupor, and visual disturbances. Seizures are the most common presenting symptom. Renal failure, malignant hypertension, autoimmune disorders, and eclampsia are common causes. The underlying pathophysiology is unknown. The goal of care is to treat the underlying cause. Hydrocephalus, permanent neurological deficit, coma, and death are complications that can occur if treatment is not administered promptly.

68. D: Eating foods rich in folic acid, such as oranges, spinach, and garbanzo beans, as well as taking a folic acid supplement prior to pregnancy, is the best way to help prevent spina bifida. Spina bifida is a neural tube defect caused by folate deficiency. It appears at conception; waiting until after

discovery of the pregnancy is too late. Most people should be ingesting 400 mcg/day of folate. Women who are pregnant, women who are trying to become pregnant, or nursing women should be ingesting 800 mcg.

69. B: ADEM is an immune-mediated inflammatory demyelinating condition that typically resolves with aggressive steroid administration. If treated quickly and appropriately, there are generally no sequelae. ADEM is usually seen in children following a viral infection or administration of a vaccine. MS is a chronic relapsing remitting immune-mediated inflammatory demyelinating condition primarily seen in the third and fifth decades of life. Steroids as well as other immunosuppressive agents can be used to treat MS flares.

70. C: This patient has 4 risk factors: obesity, history of cocaine abuse, hypertension, and sickle cell anemia. Males tender to have a higher rate for strokes than females. Other risk factors include advancing age, hyperlipidemia, diabetes, family history of stroke, race, ethnicity, alcohol abuse, and sedentary lifestyle.

71. B: The patient's advanced age, African American race, and male sex are his non-modifiable risk factors. A family history of stroke would also be considered a non-modifiable risk factor. His modifiable risk factors are tobacco abuse, hypertension, diabetes, and hyperlipidemia. Although hypertension and hyperlipidemia are not listed as part of his medical history, his blood pressure and LDL are well into the abnormal range. Normal blood pressure should be equal to or less than 130/80 mm Hg, and LDL should be less than 100 mg/dL. Other modifiable risk factors include drinking or drug abuse, obesity, sedentary lifestyle, poor diet, sickle cell anemia, polycythemia vera, renal failure, malignancy, atrial fibrillation, and heart failure.

72. B: The India ink test is the confirmatory test for cryptococcal infections. *Cryptococcus* is a fungus primarily seen in opportunistic infections in immunocompromised patients. The Western blot can be used as a confirmatory test for HIV, Creutzfeldt-Jakob disease, and hepatitis B. Rapid plasma reagin (RPR) can be used as a screening test to detect syphilis. The test is sensitive, but not specific. False-positives can occur in those who have or who have had Epstein-Barr, hepatitis, varicella, and measles. If the screening test is positive, a confirmatory test will need to be ordered. The monospot test is used to detect the Epstein-Barr virus.

73. B: In cases of viral meningitis, the protein level will be elevated due to destruction of cells (both pathogens and leukocytes). The WBC will be high due to the body trying to ward off an infection. The CSF appearance is usually clear. The CSF is usually purulent in cases of bacterial meningitis.

74. C: Strokes can present in different ways, but the most common signs and symptoms are facial droop, pronator drift, asymmetric weakness, dysarthria, preferential gaze, numbness or paresthesia in the affected extremity, and ataxia. The symptoms in choice 'a' are the triad for normal pressure hydrocephalus. The symptoms listed in choice 'b' are common signs/symptoms for acoustic neuroma. Choice 'd' describes a presentation most consistent with Parkinson disease.

75. A: The dose should be increased since the INR in subtherapeutic. The goal INR in a patient with a stroke is 2 to 3. Increasing the warfarin dose to 8 mg is too aggressive. Slow adjustments should be made to dosages to help prevent complications. Decreasing or maintaining the same dose is inappropriate since the INR is subtherapeutic.

76. D: A swallow evaluation needs to be checked first. Aspiration is a common complication is stroke patients. If the patient fails, a Dobhoff or nasogastric tube can be placed so the patient can receive medications and tube feeds.

77. B: Raising the head of the bed 30 degrees is the best initial intervention for those with high ICP. Raising the bed prevents venous blood obstruction and improves drainage, which helps to lower the ICP. Normal ICP range is 0 to 20 mm Hg. Persistently elevated ICP can cause stroke, seizure, permanent neurologic deficit, coma, and death. Although flushing the EVD and administering mannitol, a powerful osmotic diuretic, may lower ICP, these would not be the initial interventions.

78. A: The full effects of a stroke are not seen until 6 to 8 months, and sometimes longer, after the stroke. If a patient has dysarthria upon discharge, it may get better or stay the same. There is no guarantee that symptoms will improve. Family and caretakers must be made aware that the neurologic deficits may be permanent, even if the stroke that occurred is relatively small.

79. A: The patient should ambulate with assistance, at least in the beginning, to prevent injury. A patient with a traumatic brain injury may have balance issues, impulsive behavior, visual impairment, or other issues, and needs to be monitored closely when out of bed.

80. D: Performing a swallow evaluation is the least important task. It can be done after the neurological workup has been completed. Time is of the essence in the setting of a possible acute stroke. The more time that elapses, the more brain cells die and the less efficacious treatment will be.

81. C: Giving an anticonvulsant in a patient with a chronic bleed with no history of seizure is not indicated. The highest risk for seizure is in the first 1 to 2 weeks following the event. Chronic bleeds are defined as occurring 4 or more weeks following the event.

82. C: A concussion is the most common type of head injury. It can occur with open and closed head injuries. A concussion is a contusion or bruise on the brain following blunt or penetrating head trauma. It may or may not show up on radiography. Common complaints include headache, nausea, vomiting, dizziness, and loss of consciousness. The severity of the concussion determines how long it may take to heal and if any neurological deficits occur.

83. B: High-dose steroids as well as immunosuppressive therapy are the mainstays of treatment for multiple sclerosis (MS) flares. Multiple sclerosis is an autoimmune disease in which the body attacks the myelin sheath of nerve cells. Incidence peaks in the third and fifth decades. Symptoms may include slurred speech, trouble with coordination or balance, visual changes, extremity weakness, or numbness/paresthesia.

84. B: The loss of dopamine due to the destruction of the substantia nigra is responsible for Parkinson disease. One of dopamine's functions is control over smooth, purposeful movement. Some signs and symptoms of Parkinson disease include ataxia, resting tremor, muscle rigidity, mask-like facies, monotone voice, bradycardia, and hypotension.

85. A: Prions are responsible for Creutzfeldt-Jakob disease (CJD). CJD is a fatal progressive degenerative disorder caused by prions, or infectious proteins that cause normal proteins to change to an abnormal shape. They attack brain tissue, causing multiple holes in the parenchyma (also called spongiform encephalopathy).

86. A: Lewy bodies can be found in the brains of patients with dementia, as well as those with Parkinson disease. Lewy bodies are abnormal protein deposits inside of neurons. They impair the function of healthy neurons and eventually cause neuronal death.

87. D: This patient has Parkinson disease. Levodopa changes into dopamine in the brain, helping to control movement. Carbidopa prevents the breakdown of levodopa in the bloodstream so more levodopa can enter the brain.

88. A: The patient is undergoing the second emotional stage of the Kübler-Ross model. According to this model, people undergo 5 emotional stages when dealing with grief: denial, anger, bargaining, depression, and acceptance. As long as the patient's family member does not become violent with the staff, there is no reason to call the police.

89. B: Phenytoin is the best initial drug for this patient, and most commonly used to treat acute seizure activity. Levetiracetam is primarily used as maintenance therapy. Ethosuximide is primarily used for absence seizures. Pentobarbital is a short-acting barbituate used as a preanesthetic medication to help control status epilepticus. In high doses it is used for euthanasia. Since the patient only had 1 seizure and is protecting his own airway, this drug would be inappropriate.

90. A: Craniopharyngiomas generally occur near the pituitary gland of the hypothalamus. They are rare benign tumors that primarily occur in children. There are no known risk factors. Treatment is surgical resection.

91. C: Huntington disease is an autosomal dominant neurodegenerative disorder primarily seen in the fourth decade of life, although symptoms may occur any time in one's lifespan. Signs and symptoms include changes in personality, cognition, and physical skills, leading to dementia, chorea, malnutrition, sleep disturbances, seizures, ataxia, and eventually death.

92. C: The patient's lesion is likely located in the right frontal cortex. The frontal cortex controls behavior inhibition, personality, and emotion. The brain has ipsilateral control over the body; since the patient is displaying left-sided symptoms, the lesion will be located on the right side.

93. A: The patient has neurosyphilis, which is caused by *Treponema pallidum.* The mainstay of treatment is intravenous penicillin. The antibiotic will halt the progression of the disease, but will not reverse existing neurological deficits. A patient may have untreated syphilis for 10 to 20 years before developing neurosyphilis.

94. D: A lumbar puncture can be performed if a CT head without contrast is negative. A CT angiogram is the best confirmatory test, but not all hospitals may be able to perform a CT angiogram. Red blood cell count is supposed to decrease with each successive vial of cerebrospinal fluid drawn. If the red blood cell count does not change, it is diagnostic for a subarachnoid hemorrhage.

95. B: Calcium channel blockers have some selectivity for cerebral vasculature. Nimodipine is most commonly used for aneurysmal subarachnoid hemorrhage. Nimodipine's main indication is in the prevention of cerebral vasospasm and resultant ischemia.

96. C: This patient has cutaneous neurofibroma, which is an autosomal dominant malignancy that originates in the nerves of the skin. It typically appears during teenage years and progress throughout adulthood with symptoms ranging from mild to severely disfiguring.

97. C: Bell palsy causes facial asymmetry, weakness, and sometimes permanent neurologic deficit, but it is not related to stroke or transient ischemic attack. Those who present with facial numbness, weakness, and facial droop and whose workup is negative are diagnosed with Bell palsy. The etiology is unknown, but may be related to a recent herpes infection. Steroids are the mainstay of treatment, but permanent alteration in taste, facial asymmetry, or weakness may be permanent.

98. D: A mother who is experiencing a symptomatic outbreak of genital herpes (HSV-2) and delivers vaginally significantly increases the risk of the baby developing herpes encephalitis. In the event that an outbreak occurs prior to deliver, a cesarean section should be performed.

99. B: The baby is a victim of shaken baby syndrome. None of the other options cause retinal hemorrhages or subdural hematomas. Subdural hematomas are most commonly caused by trauma.

100. A: An elevated prolactin level about twice baseline is fairly predictive of a seizure. Pseudoseizure is not diagnosed with one lab value or one test. The diagnosis is based on multiple factors: a normal prolactin level, atypical symptom presentation, and clinical suspicion of nonepileptic activity are all part of the diagnostic criteria.

101. A: It is not appropriate or professional for the medical provider to confront the child's parent. The parent may not be the person responsible for the abuse. If the parent is responsible for the abuse, it is the responsibility of the police and DYFS to confront the assailant.

102. C: Sedative medications can make the patient even more confused and may increase the risk of fall. Sedatives may also cause a drop in blood pressure, which may worsen upon standing.

103. D: Hemangioblastomas arise from endothelial cells and are due to chromosomal mutations. The treatment of choice is surgery. The prognosis is generally good and recurrence is relatively uncommon.

104. C: Intravenous phenytoin can cause severe hypotension and should always be given to a patient who is on telemetry monitoring. Oral phenytoin has a significantly lower risk of cardiopulmonary complication. In the event the refractory hypotension occurs, the drug should be infused at a reduced rate or discontinued and substituted with another antiepileptic drug.

105. A: Friedreich ataxia is an autosomal recessive disorder that results in destruction of the myelin sheath of sensory neurons in the central nervous system. It primarily affects children and young adults. It is a progressive disorder. Patients eventually require the need for a wheelchair. Signs and symptoms include balance and coordination difficulties, muscle weakness, scoliosis, pes cavus, and cardiac abnormalities.

106. B: Phenytoin can cause reversible peripheral neuropathy and should be avoided when possible. Once the drug is discontinued, the peripheral neuropathy resolves.

107. D: Blood glucose should always be checked in patients that are lethargic. While serum glucose may take up to an hour to result, a fingerstick can result in less than a minute. A patient should remain NPO until all tests and labs have resulted. Feeding a patient who may need surgical

intervention increases their risk for aspiration while under anesthesia. A CRP is a nonspecific marker of inflammation and is not particularly useful in the initial workup. The patient is lethargic, but awake enough to follow commands and does not need to be intubated at this point.

108. D: The brainstem also controls life-supporting autonomic functions of the peripheral nervous system. Even small abnormalities that occur in this area have devastating effects on the patient.

109. D: The husband is confused and lethargic, and is not reliable. The wife can relay whether or not he lost consciousness, which may give better insight to the extent of his injury.

110. C: The patient's GCS is 12. The patient's best eye response is a 3, best verbal response is a 4, and best motor response is a 5.

# Glasgow Coma Scale

| | | |
|---|---|---|
| Best eye response (E) | Spontaneous--open with blinking at baseline | 4 |
| | Opens to verbal command, speech, or shout | 3 |
| | Opens to pain, not applied to face | 2 |
| | None | 1 |
| Best verbal response (V) | Oriented | 5 |
| | Confused conversation, but able to answer questions | 4 |
| | Inappropriate responses, words discernible | 3 |
| | Incomprehensible speech | 2 |
| | None | 1 |
| Best motor response (M) | Obeys commands for movement | 6 |
| | Purposeful movement to painful stimulus | 5 |
| | Withdraws from pain | 4 |
| | Abnormal (spastic) flexion, decorticate posture | 3 |
| | Extensor (rigid) response, decerebrate posture | 2 |
| | None | 1 |

111. A: Cheyne–Stokes breathing is an abnormal occurrence seen in those with brainstem injuries, neonates, and those with chronic heart failure. Periods of apnea lead to increased carbon dioxide, which causes excessive hyperventilation. Hyperventilation causes carbon dioxide levels to plummet, which causes apnea, restarting the cycle.

112. B: This patient has a battle sign that is indicative of a basilar fracture. It is a rare fracture consistent with severe trauma. Patients may present with raccoon eyes (infraorbital ecchymoses) or battle sign(s).

113. D: Pentobarbital is a short-acting barbiturate used as a preanesthetic medication to help control status epilepticus. It slows the activity of the brain and nervous system. It should not be

used for initial management of seizure. Intravenous antiepileptic drugs, benzodiazepines, and amnestic agents such as propofol (Diprivan) infusions should be attempted first.

114. A: The Jacksonian march is typically seen with simple partial seizures. It is a progression of the location of the seizure in the brain, which leads to a "march" of the motor presentation of symptoms.

115. A: Benzodiazepines such as lorazepam (Ativan) are typically given with antiepileptic drugs. They are quicker acting than antiepileptic drugs and have proven efficacy at terminating seizure activity. If intravenous administration is difficult, many benzodiazepines can be given via the intramuscular route.

116. C: Having the patient lie in the lateral recumbent position during a seizure significantly reduces the risk of aspiration. Being on one's side allows debris and fluid to fall out of the mouth and prevents the tongue from blocking the airway.

117. D: Pseudoseizure is not diagnosed with one lab value or one test. The diagnosis is based on multiple factors: a normal prolactin level, atypical symptom presentation, and clinical suspicion of nonepileptic activity are all part of the diagnostic criteria. The patient displays eye-rolling and generalized body tremors, but remains awake and alert, which is a highly unusual presentation. Grand mal seizures are usually preceded by an aura, progress to a loss of consciousness, eye-rolling, tongue biting, generalized tremors, and incontinence, followed by a postictal period.

118. B: Blindness is not a complication of basilar skull fractures. Since the location of the fracture is by the temporal area, hearing complications are the most common deficit.

119. D: Avoidance of blowing the nose, coughing vigorously, and straining are typical recommendations given to those who have a skull fracture. These types of actions may further tear the meninges. Although it is a rare occurrence, bacteria can enter these tears and cause infection.

120. B: The patient's neurological exam is significantly depressed; the patient should be intubated immediately for airway protection. Generally, patients with a GCS less than 8 should be intubated. CT of the brain can be done once the airway is secured. Blood work can be drawn en route to CT scan. If peripheral access cannot be obtained, then intraosseous (IO) access can be obtained in the ER and a central line can be placed later.

121. B: Due to HIPAA (Health Insurance Portability and Accountability Act), a patient's right to privacy should be protected. There is no way to verify the identity of this person over the telephone so no information regarding the patient should be given. The person can be offered a chance to come to the hospital so staff can confirm the identity.

122. B: Giving aspirin per rectum is the best course of action in this patient, even though he arrived in the ER within the tPA window. New research found that tPA can be given up to 4.5 hours after known symptom onset. However, due to the size of the stroke seen on CT scan in combination with the patient's advanced age and incredibly high NIHSS score, aspirin would be the wisest choice. The patient is at very high risk for hemorrhagic conversion. His overall prognosis is poor.

123. B: Atherosclerosis is the most common cause of thrombotic strokes. The narrowed lumen of the vasculature causes slowing of blood flow, which promotes clot formation. Thrombotic strokes are the most common type of stroke.

124. B: The patient is severely neurologically depressed with no signs of improvement for the past week. The family should be approached about making the patient comfort measures only. Brain death protocol should only be performed if there are no brainstem reflexes present and the family refuses to withdraw care. Since this patient's GCS is a 5, some brainstem reflexes are still present.

125. C: This patient has Tourette syndrome. This condition is characterized by involuntary motor tics and or verbalizations. It generally starts in childhood. There are many medications available to help control the symptoms. Motor seizures would involve involuntary tremors. Tardive dyskinesia is an involuntary abnormal movement of the tongue.

126. A: Ropinirole (Requip) is a medication used to treat Parkinson disease and RLS. RLS is characterized by painful or uncomfortable sensations in the legs, particularly at night. Movement helps alleviate the discomfort. The underlying etiology is unknown. Labetalol and esmolol are beta-blockers; they play no role in the treatment of RLS. Haloperidol is an antipsychotic medication that is not used to treat RLS.

127. C: Those with sleep apnea are at risk for stroke. Obstructive sleep apnea predisposes to cardiac arrhythmias such as paroxysmal atrial fibrillation. This can cause a cardioembolic stroke.

128. D: Becoming a patient's sponsor should be left to a substance abuse counselor. These specialists can be found at substance support groups referred by a social worker.

129. A: Seizures due to alcohol withdrawal are a common occurrence and this patient should be closely monitored while in the hospital. Patients do not need to be put on prophylactic anticonvulsant medications. The patient should be placed on benzodiazepine therapy as well as a banana bag.

130. D: This patient has neurocysticercosis, a parasitic infection caused by eating contaminated or uncooked pork. The most common presenting symptom is seizure. It is primarily seen in third world countries. The proteinaceous material from the larvae rupturing from their cysts and the calcifications caused by dead parasites cause obstructive hydrocephalus. Patients often require a ventricular peritoneal shunt (VPS), which may repeatedly get clogged due to the calcifications and protein debris.

131. B: Intracranial hemorrhage, recent head trauma in the last 3 months, active internal bleeding, uncontrolled blood pressure (more than 185/100 mm Hg), abnormal clotting factors due to malignancy or anticoagulation (INR more than 1.7, platelet count less than 100,000/mm³), glucose less than 50 mg/dL or more than 400 mg/dL, and seizure at stroke onset are other absolute contraindications to tPA. Relative contraindications include rapidly improving or resolved symptoms, major surgery/trauma (excluding head trauma) within 2 weeks, GI or GU bleed within 3 weeks, pregnancy, recent lumbar puncture, recent arterial stick at a noncompressible site, and history of myocarditis or pericarditis.

132. D: TPA can be used only in those who are 18 years and older. The newest guidelines show that it can be used up to 4.5 hours after symptom onset; however, it should be administered as soon as possible to increase the chance of improvement. Pregnancy is a relative contraindication for tPA. One of the major complications of tPA is hemorrhagic conversion.

133. C: Arrhythmic contractions of the heart increase the likelihood of clot formation, which travels from the heart to the brain causing a stroke. A 2D echocardiogram should be part of every stroke workup to rule out cardioembolic source.

134. A: Rhabdoid tumors are highly malignant tumors that most frequently occur in infants and young children. They are generally found in the cerebral hemispheres. Due to age, radiation therapy is not an option. The mainstays of treatment are chemotherapy and tumor debulking. These options are generally palliative since the prognosis is very poor (mean survival rate is less than 2 years).

135. B: Osteosarcoma is the most common form of bone malignancy. They most commonly occur in children and young adults. The most common locations are the proximal tibia and the distal femur. Mainstays of therapy are surgical resection and chemotherapy. Amputation may sometimes be needed. Osteochondromas are benign tumors of the bone. Chordomas and malignant giant cell tumors are rare primary bone malignancies.

136. D: Haloperidol is an antipsychotic drug and plays no role in the treatment of multiple sclerosis.

137. C: Breast cancer most commonly metastasizes to the bone. Lung and prostate cancers also frequently spread to the bone.

138. C: This patient has a subacute subdural hematoma. Acute bleeds occur 1 to 2 weeks following an injury. Subacute bleeds occur 2 to 4 weeks following an injury. Chronic bleeds occur more than 4 weeks following an injury. Acute on chronic bleeds have components of acute blood within a chronic bleed.

139. A: Discontinue the tPA. Seizure before or during tPA administration is an absolute contraindication. Once the tPA has been discontinued, anticonvulsant drugs can be given and an EEG can be placed. As long as the vitals remain stable and the patient does not develop status epilepticus, the patient does not need to be intubated.

140. B: Rhabdoid tumors are highly malignant tumors that most frequently occur in infants and young children. Macrocephaly, seizure, and coordination and balance difficulties are common presenting symptoms. This malignancy is generally found in the cerebral hemispheres. Due to age, radiation therapy is not an option. The mainstays of treatment are chemotherapy and tumor debulking. These options are generally palliative since the prognosis is very poor (mean survival rate is less than 2 years).

141. B: Females, African Americans, tobacco abuse, hypertension, family history, and history of previous cerebral aneurysms are all risk factors for developing an aneurysm.

142. D: Optic neuritis is highly associated with multiple sclerosis. In some people, signs and symptoms of optic neuritis may be the first indication of multiple sclerosis. Signs and symptoms include flashing or flickering lights, decreased ability to see color saturation, and dull aching pain. It is caused by temporary inflammation of the optic nerve. Steroids are the mainstay of treatment.

143. C: Even though the patient's symptoms resolved, they should be kept at least overnight so a stroke workup can be done. All labs and radiological findings should be resulted prior to discharge and a neurologist should be consulted.

144. C: Vasospasm causes narrowing of a cerebral blood vessel and reduced blood flow. This may lead to delayed ischemia and cerebral infarction if left untreated. The mainstay of treatment for aneurysmal SAH is triple H therapy: hypertension, hypervolemia, and hemodilution.

145. A: An acoustic neuroma is an uncommon benign tumor that develops on the eighth cranial nerve. Common signs and symptoms include hearing changes, balance difficulties, vertigo, and facial weakness. Neurofibromatosis is the only known risk factor.

146. B: Decorticate posture severe traumatic injury. It is a sign of damage to the nerve pathway between the brain and spinal cord.

147. A: The patient should be sitting up with the head of bed at 30 degrees or have the patient lie in the lateral recumbent position. These positions are optimal to help prevent aspiration.

148. C: A relative contraindication to tPA is minor or rapidly improving symptoms. Since the NIHSS is so low, giving aspirin only is the best course of action. Warfarin does not play a role in the setting of acute stroke or transient ischemic attack. Not giving any medications is inappropriate for this patient.

149. C: Knowing the symptom onset is crucial information. Tissue plasminogen activator (tPA) can be given up to 4.5 hours after symptom onset. If the time onset is unknown, tPA will not be able to be administered and the patient could lose out on a potential life-saving medical intervention.

150. D: The MAP is the most crucial vital sign. Permissive hypertension in the 24-hour period following a stroke is important to maintain brain perfusion. This will help salvage the area of penumbra. However, if the MAP becomes too high, the patient will be at risk for hemorrhagic conversion.

151. B: The motor assessment as well as the patient's speech and mentation are important aspects to monitor. If the neurological exam changes, the provider should order a stat CT of the brain to monitor the patient for possible hemorrhagic conversion.

152. A: Warfarin as well as beta-blockers and antiarrhythmic medications such as digoxin (Lanoxin) would be prescribed for this patient. Atrial fibrillation increases the risk for stroke fourfold so this condition needs to be strictly controlled. Arrhythmic contractions of the heart increase the likelihood of clot formation, which travels from the heart to the brain causing a stroke. Blood thinners such as warfarin prevent these clots from forming.

153. A: African Americans and males are the highest risk groups for stroke. His cocaine abuse is also a significant risk factor. Factors such as hypertension, diabetes, obesity, sickle cell disease, tobacco abuse, and atrial fibrillation also increase the risk for stroke. Women and Asians generally are at lower risk. Chronic anemia is not a significant risk factor.

154. D: Decerebrate posturing is an abnormal body posture that involves the arms and legs being held straight out and the toes are pointed downward. This is an ominous finding for severe brain damage. The prognosis is very poor.

155. D: The serum glucose is an absolute contraindication to thrombolytics. The patient should receive antiplatelet therapy instead. Intracranial hemorrhage, recent head trauma in the last 3 months, active internal bleeding, uncontrolled blood pressure (more than 185/100 mm Hg),

abnormal clotting factors due to malignancy or anticoagulation (INR more than 1.7, platelet count less than 100,000/mm³), glucose less than 50 mg/dL or more than 400 mg/dL, and seizure at stroke onset are other absolute contraindications to tPA. Relative contraindications include rapidly improving or resolved symptoms, major surgery/trauma (excluding head trauma) within 2 weeks, GI or GU bleed within 3 weeks, pregnancy, recent lumbar puncture, recent arterial stick at a noncompressible site, and history of myocarditis or pericarditis.

156. A: Encouraging the patient to feed himself is not particularly helpful. In addition to his motor deficits, the patient may also have dysphagia and cognitive deficits that would impair him further.

157. B: A patient who is having difficulty with rapidly touching their own nose and then touching the examiner's finger (or any form of rapidly alternating movement) is called dysmetria. It is a sign of cerebellar dysfunction.

158. B: The patient is at risk for decubitus ulcers and having a family member inspect the skin for signs of reddening or breakdown illustrates that he understands how to care for the patient. The other actions place the patient at risk of fall or aspiration.

159. C: This patient has a dystrophic gait. Helicopod gait is when the patient takes a step and rotates in a small half circle. Ataxic gait is staggering or stumbling gait. Parkinsonian gait is characterized by slow, shuffling movements.

160. C: Dropping saline drops in the patient's eyes or using a cotton-tipped applicator to touch the eyes will help assess corneal reflexes. Even patients who are comatose can blink when stimuli is applied to the eye. The loss of this reflex shows significant brainstem dysfunction.

161. B: Females are at lower risk for stroke than males. African Americans and Latinos are the highest risk groups for stroke. Factors such as hypertension, diabetes, obesity, sickle cell disease, tobacco abuse, and atrial fibrillation also increase the risk for stroke.

162. D: If the patient is claustrophobic, they will need a benzodiazepine prior to MRI. Since the patient will be lying flat and is likely lethargic, feeding the patient prior to the test increases the risk of aspiration.

163. D: The best initial intervention is to redirect the patient's behavior. It is the least invasive form of intervention. If that fails, the patient may require a 1:1 safety watch and possibly restraints if their behavior poses a threat to themselves or to staff. A psychiatry consult would be warranted if the patient's behavior is refractory to all other measures.

164. D: The goal of treatment is to eliminate carbon dioxide. That is because an acid environment in the brain causes cerebral vessels to dilate and therefore increases ICP.

165. B: Most patients with permanent pacemakers cannot undergo MRIs because the magnetic and radiofrequency fields may cause the pacemaker to stop functioning. Also, because the pacemaker is metal, there is risk for traumatic removal from the patient's chest. Cataract surgery, gallbladder surgery, and vasectomies are not contraindications for MRI. The surgical clips used in cholecystectomy procedures do not pose a problem with MRIs.

# Practice Test #2

## Practice Questions

1. A patient with a known seizure disorder is admitted to the hospital with altered mental status. His phenytoin (Dilantin) level is 35.6. What is the most appropriate action?
    a. Bolus with 1 gram of phenytoin.
    b. Continue to give the patient's standard dosage of phenytoin.
    c. Hold phenytoin and recheck a level the next day.
    d. Administer naloxone (Narcan).

2. Which of the following are sources of an embolic stroke?
    a. Hypertension.
    b. Patent foramen ovale.
    c. Obesity.
    d. Hyperlipidemia.

3. A patient complaining of a headache for the past several weeks is diagnosed with a subacute subdural hematoma. Which of the following is not an appropriate course of action?
    a. Repeat CT of the head.
    b. Administer acetaminophen (Tylenol).
    c. Serial neurological assessments.
    d. Administer levetiracetam (Keppra).

4. Which of the following regarding astrocytomas is not correct?
    a. Grade IV astrocytomas are benign.
    b. Astrocytomas arise from astrocytes.
    c. Chemotherapy and radiation are common treatments.
    d. Astrocytoma is the most common glioma.

5. A patient is diagnosed with amyotrophic lateral sclerosis (ALS) and the patient's wife is concerned about their children developing this condition. Which of the following is an appropriate response?
    a. It is an x-linked chromosomal disease.
    b. It is an autosomal dominant disease.
    c. It is an autosomal recessive disease.
    d. Its etiology is unknown.

6. A patient presents with unilateral sharp, throbbing headaches associated with eye pain and watering. What is the most likely diagnosis?
    a. Cluster headache.
    b. Trigeminal neuralgia.
    c. Tension headache.
    d. Fibromyalgia.

7. A child is born with dozens café-au-lait spots and axillary freckling. What is the most likely diagnosis?
    a. Hemangioblastoma.
    b. Meningioma.
    c. Neurofibromatosis.
    d. Craniopharyngioma.

8. A child with spina bifida develops worsening headaches and visual problems. An MRI of the brain reveals herniation of the brainstem and lower part of the cerebellum extending into the foramen magnum. Which type of Chiari malformation does this condition describe?
    a. Type I.
    b. Type II.
    c. Type III.
    d. Type IV.

9. Which of the following is the most common presenting symptom for Chiari malformation?
    a. Facial palsy.
    b. Resting tremor.
    c. Ascending weakness.
    d. Occipital headaches.

10. A patient presenting with dysarthria and lethargy is being evaluated in the ER for possible stroke. The patient has a Glasgow Coma Scale (GCS) of 12, blood pressure of 150/72, pulse ox of 96% on room air, blood glucose of 43, and patient scores a 9 on the National Institutes of Health Stroke Scale (NIHSS). What is the best next step in intervention?
    a. Administer D50.
    b. Obtain a CT of the head.
    c. Administer tissue plasminogen activator (tPA).
    d. Intubate the patient.

11. Which of the following is true regarding multiple sclerosis (MS)?
    a. MS is an autoimmune disease.
    b. MS is more common in people indigenous to the tropics.
    c. MS affects men more than women.
    d. MS can be cured with steroids.

12. Which of the following conditions involves chronic widespread pain and a heightened response to pressure?
    a. Multiple sclerosis.
    b. Amyotrophic Lateral Sclerosis.
    c. Fibromyalgia.
    d. Guillain-Barré syndrome.

13. An 89-year-old female suffers a mechanical fall and presents to the hospital complaining of back pain. A MRI of the lumbar spine reveals an acute L1 compression fracture without retropulsion into the spinal canal or impingement of the spinal cord. The patient has no neurologic deficits. Which of the following would be the least appropriate initial step in management?
   a. Steroid injections.
   b. Diskectomy and fusion.
   c. Physical therapy.
   d. Lumbar sacral orthotic (LSO) brace.

14. Which of the following conditions would be an unlikely etiology of a brain abscess?
   a. Acquired immune deficiency syndrome (AIDS).
   b. Calvarial fracture.
   c. Sinusitis.
   d. Guillain-Barré syndrome (GBS).

15. A patient developed sudden onset right hemiparesis and facial droop one hour prior to arrival in the emergency room. The patient had a tonic-clonic seizure at the time of symptom onset, which spontaneously resolved without medication. The patient's labs and CT of the head are normal. The patient is lethargic, but following commands. The National Institutes of Health Stroke Scale (NIHSS) is fifteen. Which of the following is the next step in management?
   a. Intubate the patient.
   b. Administer tissue plasminogen activator (tPA).
   c. Discharge the patient home.
   d. Obtain an electroencephalogram (EEG).

16. Which of the following statements about trigeminal neuralgia (TGN) are true? (Select all that apply).
   a. TGN is caused by compression of the seventh cranial nerve.
   b. Anticonvulsant medicines are generally effective in treating TGN.
   c. Women are more commonly affected than men.
   d. TGN flare–ups generally occur at night.

17. A woman is trying to conceive and is concerned about her child being born with spina bifida. The patient should be encouraged to eat more of which of the following foods? (Select all that apply).
   a. Garbanzo beans (chickpeas).
   b. Collard greens.
   c. Oranges.
   d. Garlic.

18. A patient complains of burning painful rash on the right side of her trunk for the past four months. On exam the patient has intact vesicles on an erythematous base in a band on the right lower trunk. Which of the following is the most likely etiology?
   a. Varicella zoster.
   b. Rubella.
   c. Rubeola.
   d. Epstein-Barr virus.

19. A patient status post motor vehicle accident is being evaluated at the bedside. The patient is intubated, his eyes open to sternal rub, and he withdraws to noxious stimuli. What is his Glasgow Coma Scale (GCS)?
   a. Five.
   b. Six.
   c. Seven.
   d. Eight.

20. A patient develops progressively worsening low back pain over several months. The pain is alleviated with rest. There are no other associated symptoms. Which of the following is the most likely diagnosis?
   a. Epidural abscess.
   b. Herniated nucleus pulposus.
   c. Epidural tumor.
   d. Meningitis.

21. A patient is diagnosed with carpal tunnel syndrome. Impingement on which of the following causes this condition?
   a. Radial nerve.
   b. Median nerve.
   c. Trigeminal nerve.
   d. Ulnar nerve.

22. A patient diagnosed with whiplash is being discharged from the hospital. Which of the following recommendations regarding the treatment of whiplash are correct? (Select all that apply).
   a. Wear a cervical collar all day except when showering.
   b. Use NSAIDs as needed.
   c. Lidocaine injections may provide relief.
   d. Apply ice or heat to the neck several times a day.

23. A patient receives an epidural prior to the birth of her child. She develops a cerebrospinal fluid (CSF) leak following the procedure. Which of the following interventions may alleviate her symptoms? (Select all that apply).
   a. Blood patch.
   b. Increasing her fluid intake.
   c. NSAIDs.
   d. Reverse Trendelenburg position.

24. A child is brought to the hospital with high fever, lethargy, and new onset seizure. The child is diagnosed with meningitis. The mother reports that her child is not vaccinated. Which of the following is the most likely etiology for the child's illness?
   a. *Cryptococcus.*
   b. *Neisseria meningitides.*
   c. *Listeria monocytogenes.*
   d. *Haemophilus influenza.*

25. A patient is brought to the hospital after being struck in the head with a bat. The patient's Glasgow Coma Scale is thirteen. A CT scan of the head reveals a nondisplaced parietal fracture and with hypodense convexity in the right parietal area. There is no blunting of the ventricles. Which of the following is not an appropriate intervention?
    a. Prepare the patient for a craniotomy.
    b. Insert an intraventricular drain.
    c. Administer an antiepileptic drug.
    d. Perform serial neurological exams.

26. A patient is diagnosed with benign paroxysmal positional vertigo (BPPV). She inquires how she can prevent future flare-ups. Which of the following is a correct response? (Select all that apply).
    a. Decrease fluid intake.
    b. Avoid sudden or rapid body movements.
    c. Drinking red wine several times a week may alleviate symptoms.
    d. Avoid sleeping on the affected side.

27. Which of the following are major contraindications for tissue plasminogen activator (tPA)? (Select all that apply).
    a. Blood pressure 200/120.
    b. INR 2.5.
    c. Recent head trauma in the last year.
    d. Serum glucose 60 mg/dL.

28. Which of the following conditions is included in Cushing's triad?
    a. Irregular respirations.
    b. Hypotension.
    c. Tachycardia.
    d. Seizure.

29. A patient flexes his head and knees when his neck is flexed. This physical finding indicates which of the following conditions?
    a. Cerebral abscess.
    b. Benign paroxysmal positional vertigo.
    c. Meningitis.
    d. Myasthenia gravis.

30. Which of the following signs/symptoms is part of the classic triad of normal pressure hydrocephalus (NPH)? (Select all that apply).
    a. Nystagmus.
    b. Dementia.
    c. Seizure.
    d. Ataxia.

31. A patient has just been diagnosed with Meniere's disease. Which of the following is the most appropriate treatment?
    a. Referral to a geneticist.
    b. Referral to an oncologist.
    c. Referral to an audiologist.
    d. Referral to palliative care.

32. A 43-year-old male from Guatemala presents with worsening back pain associated with fever, chills, fatigue, and paresthesias in his lower extremities for the past four months. He notes that he had a cough with hemoptysis, unintentional weight loss, and night sweats a year ago but was never treated. His purified protein derivative was positive. A MRI with gadolinium revealed lytic destruction of multiple vertebral bodies in his lumbar spine. Which of the following is the most likely diagnosis?
    a. Ependymoma.
    b. Chronic inflammatory demyelinating polyneuropathy.
    c. Scheuermann's disease.
    d. Pott's disease.

33. A patient is in the intensive care unit following an assault to the head. Her eyes open to pain, she is verbal but confused, and she will follow some simple commands. In terms of her motor exam, what is her Glasgow Coma Scale (GCS) score?
    a. Two.
    b. Five.
    c. Six.
    d. Thirteen.

34. Which of the following is not a treatment for a patient with an aneurysmal subarachnoid hemorrhage in vasospasm?
    a. Intravenous fluid hydration.
    b. Diuretics.
    c. Calcium channel blockers.
    d. Vasopressors.

35. A patient suffers from a sudden fall without loss of consciousness. The patient is diagnosed with a stroke. What type of stroke does the patient most likely have?
    a. Basilar.
    b. Frontal.
    c. Parietal.
    d. Thalamic.

36. Which of the following is the most likely possible complication of a basal ganglia bleed (BGB)?
    a. Blindness.
    b. Hydrocephalus.
    c. Hearing loss.
    d. Seizure.

37. A patient is diagnosed with Wernicke-Korsakoff syndrome (WKS). What is an important treatment for this condition?
    a. Antiviral medication.
    b. Steroids.
    c. Antibiotics.
    d. Thiamine.

38. Which of the following statements regarding arteriovenous malformations (AVMs) are correct? (Select all that apply).
    a. AVMs are rare conditions.
    b. AVMs most commonly occur in the brain and spine.
    c. AVMs are an autosomal recessive condition.
    d. AVMs require surgical resection.

39. A patient is diagnosed with diffuse axonal injury (DAI). Which of the following radiological findings are most consistent with this diagnosis?
    a. Hypodense convexity.
    b. Enlargement of the temporal horns of the lateral ventricles.
    c. Punctuate hypodensities and cerebral edema.
    d. Hypodense concavity.

40. A 68-year-old male patient is admitted to the hospital for an acute lacunar infarct. His only known medical problem is iron deficiency anemia, but he has not been seen by a primary care physician in sixteen years. In the ER the patient's admission labs and vital signs are as follows: BP 175/99, EKG shows sinus bradycardia with a heart rate of 45 bpm, HA1c is 8.8%, Na 145, K 4.1, Cl 100, CO2, 30, BUN 19, Cr 1.2, glucose 386, LDL 155, HDL 38, cholesterol 251, WBC 10.1, hemoglobin 12.4, hematocrit 38.5, platelets 258,000. How many risk factors did this patient have for developing a stroke?
    a. 3.
    b. 4.
    c. 5.
    d. 6.

41. Which of the following would most likely be associated with an acute occipital lobe stroke?
    a. Vision loss.
    b. Flat affect.
    c. Fluent aphasia.
    d. Impulsive inhibition difficulty.

42. A patient with a known history of renal cell carcinoma develops worsening headaches and confusion. A MRI of the brain reveals half a dozen bilateral brain metastases. Which of the following is not a likely intervention?
    a. Surgical removal of the brain lesions.
    b. Oral steroids.
    c. Radiation therapy.
    d. Anticonvulsant drugs.

43. A 16-year-old patient presents with recurrent seizure-like activity over the past month. She has history of depression and obesity. She has no known recent head trauma or cerebral infection. During her episodes she displays generalized tonic clonic activity, but is able to continue a conversation with her examiner. What would be the next step in management? (Select all that apply).
    a. Order a bolus of Dilantin.
    b. Obtain an electroencephalogram (EEG).
    c. Obtain a prolactin level.
    d. Order a psychiatry consult.

44. What is the primary treatment of metastatic spinal tumors?
    a. Surgical repair.
    b. Chemotherapy.
    c. Orthotic brace.
    d. Radiation.

45. During a physical assessment the examiner has the patient hold their arms out in front of them. The patient flexes their wrists, letting their hands hang down. The examiner evaluates the patient to see if tingling, numbness, or pain in the fingers develops. What is this diagnostic test called and what condition does it indicate?
    a. Phalen maneuver, ulnar nerve entrapment.
    b. Phalen maneuver, carpal tunnel syndrome.
    c. Tinel sign, ulnar nerve entrapment.
    d. Tinel sign, carpal tunnel syndrome.

46. Which of the following tests helps diagnose benign paroxysmal positional vertigo (BPPV)?
    a. Electroencephalogram.
    b. Dix-Hallpike maneuver.
    c. Caloric stimulation.
    d. Electrocochleography.

47. Which of the following is not part of the classic triad seen with Wernicke-Korsakoff syndrome (WKS)? (Select all that apply).
    a. Bradycardia.
    b. Opthalmoplegia.
    c. Dementia.
    d. Cortical blindness.

48. What would be considered reasonable management of a patient with a nondepressed skull fracture with a Glasgow Coma Scale (GCS) of 15?
    a. Insert an external ventricular drain.
    b. Schedule a craniectomy.
    c. Follow up as an outpatient.
    d. Schedule a craniotomy.

49. A patient diagnosed with an oligodendroglioma is concerned about her lifespan and asks you about the prognosis about this condition. Which of the following is the most appropriate response?
    a. The condition is curative with aggressive chemotherapy.
    b. The condition is terminal, but patients generally die several years after symptom onset.
    c. Most patients generally die within months of the diagnosis.
    d. This is a benign condition.

50. What is the most common treatment(s) for malignant pineal tumors (germinomas)?
    a. Chemotherapy and radiation.
    b. Chemotherapy, radiation, and surgical resection.
    c. Surgical resection only.
    d. Chemotherapy only.

51. Which of the following signs and symptoms are most commonly seen with oligodendromas?
   a. Tinnitus, hearing loss, ataxia.
   b. Chorea, tardive dyskinesia, dementia.
   c. Recurrent syncopal episodes.
   d. Headache, seizure, personality changes.

52. A patient has been brought to the hospital after being struck by a car. On physical exam the patient opens his eyes to noxious stimuli, is moving spontaneously but doesn't follow commands, and is confused but responds to questions. Which of the following is the most appropriate initial intervention?
   a. Obtain a CT of the head.
   b. Intubate the patient.
   c. Administer an anti-epileptic drug.
   d. Place the patient in soft restraints.

53. During a trauma work-up a 3 mm left middle cerebral artery aneurysm is found. The patient has a known history of tobacco abuse and hypertension, but no history of known aneurysms. What is the most appropriate advice to give the patient's spouse?
   a. The patient's family members should be scanned for aneurysms.
   b. The patient will need serial imaging as an outpatient.
   c. Small aneurysms are a common incidental finding.
   d. This aneurysm will require urgent surgery.

54. Which of the following test(s) is used to help monitor vasospasm in aneurysmal subarachnoid patients? (Select all that apply).
   a. X-ray of the head
   b. MRI of the brain
   c. CT angiogram of the brain
   d. Transcranial dopplers

55. A person is diagnosed with an aneurysmal subarachnoid hemorrhage. When is the highest likelihood that this patient will develop vasospasm?
   a. 1-2 weeks.
   b. 2-3 weeks.
   c. 3-4 weeks.
   d. More than 4 weeks.

56. A patient has been diagnosed with chondrosarcoma. His wife is concerned about their children developing this condition. Which of the following is the most appropriate statement?
   a. Children will need to be tested because it is an autosomal recessive condition.
   b. Only male children will need to be tested since it is an X-linked condition.
   c. Children will not need to be tested since the etiology is unknown.
   d. The children will not seed to be tested since tobacco use is the only known risk factor.

57. Which of the following is the most common presenting symptom for a schwannoma?
   a. Tinnitus.
   b. Dementia.
   c. Personality changes.
   d. Seizure.

58. Which of the following intervention(s) is appropriate for a child with cerebral palsy (CP)? (Select all that apply).
a. Physical therapy.
b. Baclofen (Lioresal).
c. Speech therapy.
d. Phenytoin (Dilantin).

59. The destruction of which of the following neurotransmitters causes symptoms in Parkinson's disease?
a. Serotonin.
b. Norepinephrine.
c. Epinephrine.
d. Dopamine.

60. Which of the following is primarily responsible for the development of spina bifida?
a. Alcohol abuse.
b. Tobacco abuse.
c. Dietary deficiency.
d. Genetic.

61. A patient notices a unilateral upper extremity fine motor tremor that worsens with activity. It improves with rest. The patient has no other symptoms. What is the most likely diagnosis?
a. Simple motor seizure.
b. Tourette's syndrome.
c. Essential tremor.
d. Parkinson's disease.

62. Which of the following malignancies is least likely to metastasize to the brain?
a. Pancreas.
b. Lung.
c. Breast.
d. Melanoma.

63. Which of the following conditions are most likely to spread in a prison?
a. Amyotrophic lateral sclerosis.
b. Meningitis.
c. Cerebral abscess.
d. Myasthenia gravis.

64. A patient who suffered a large stroke has left hemiparesis. Which of the following interventions will help prevent future complications? (Select all that apply).
a. Frequent repositioning
b. Placement of foley catheter
c. Assisting with feeding
d. Cluster nursing interventions

65. Which of the following is the most appropriate treatment for essential tremor?
   a. Propranolol (Inderal).
   b. Baclofen (Lioresal).
   c. Levetiracetam (Keppra).
   d. Metoclopramide (Reglan).

66. Which of the following age groups is the most at risk for developing petit mal seizures?
   a. 5–10 years old.
   b. 15–20 years old.
   c. 35–40 years old.
   d. 60–65 years old.

67. A mother brings her child to the hospital after the child develops a new onset seizure. The child is found to have an ear infection. Their oral temperature is 102.1. Which of the following statements is true regarding this condition?
   a. Febrile seizures may occur in children as young as three months to six years of age.
   b. Febrile seizures usually resolve with anticonvulsants.
   c. Febrile seizures do not have a genetic component.
   d. Febrile seizures may cause some neurologic impairment.

68. A patient is diagnosed with a brainstem, stroke. Which of the following would not be affected?
   a. Respiratory rate.
   b. Blood pressure.
   c. Heart rate.
   d. Language comprehension.

69. Which of the following illustrates the most common cause of carotid dissection in young patients?
   a. A patient with a LDL of 155.
   b. A patient in a motor vehicle accident.
   c. A patient with a blood pressure of 165/112.
   d. A patient who has a history of tobacco abuse.

70. Which of the following etiologies is most likely responsible to cause a basal ganglia bleed?
   a. Motor vehicle accident.
   b. Aneurysmal rupture.
   c. Hypertension.
   d. Seizure.

71. Which of the following may trigger a seizure in patients with a known history of seizure disorder? (Select all that may apply).
   a. Stress.
   b. Alcohol.
   c. Exercise.
   d. Sleep deprivation.

72. A 2nd trimester fetus is noted to have hydrocephalus and intracranial calcifications. The mother notes having nonspecific upper respiratory symptoms a few weeks ago, but the symptoms spontaneously resolved. The mother has no significant past medical history. Upon further investigation it is discovered she keeps several cats as pets. Which of the following is the most likely cause of the fetus's findings?
    a. Cytomegalovirus.
    b. Toxoplasmosis.
    c. Syphilis.
    d. Parvovirus B19.

73. A patient is diagnosed with a parietal lobe tumor. Which of the following would not be affected?
    a. Reading.
    b. Memory.
    c. Writing.
    d. Calculations.

74. A patient has just undergone a lumbar puncture. Which of the following instructions are most appropriate to give to the patient?
    a. You should lie flat for several hours.
    b. You may drink alcohol in moderation.
    c. You should limit your fluid intake.
    d. You can resume regular activity.

75. Which of the following most accurately describes how to diagnose epilepsy?
    a. 4 or more epileptic episodes in twenty-hour hours.
    b. 2 or more epileptic episodes in twelve hours.
    c. 2 or more epileptic episodes in twenty-hour hours.
    d. 4 or more epileptic episodes in twelve hours.

76. Which of the following most accurately describes a child born with fetal alcohol syndrome (FAS)?
    a. Smooth philtrum, thin vermilion border, microcephaly.
    b. Jaundice, petechiae, hearing loss.
    c. Vesicular rash, poor feeding, seizures.
    d. Neurosensory deafness, mandibular hypoplasia, retinopathy.

77. Which of the following signs and symptoms commonly occur with pellagra?
    a. Paralysis, respiratory insufficiency, cognitive decline.
    b. Seizures, cortical blindness, developmental delay.
    c. Microcephaly, macroglossia, malnutrition.
    d. Diarrhea, dermatitis, dementia.

78. A woman gives birth to a child with anencephaly. The mother requests the prognosis for this condition. Which of the following is the most appropriate response?
    a. The prognosis is good with surgical intervention.
    b. The prognosis is guarded with surgical intervention.
    c. The child will likely have moderate motor and cognitive deficits.
    d. There is no treatment and the condition is fatal.

79. A mother with a remote history of an unknown sexually transmitted disease gives birth to an infant who develops seizure, poor feeding, temperature instability, and full fontanel. Which of the following is most likely responsible for the baby's condition?
    a. Genital warts.
    b. Herpes simplex II.
    c. Bacterial vaginosis.
    d. Chlamydia.

80. Which of the following are appropriate treatment modalities for a patient with Alzheimer's disease? (Select all that apply).
    a. Encourage frequent bathroom trips.
    b. Fill out a calendar with daily activities.
    c. Encourage bedrest.
    d. Take frequent skin assessments.

81. A patient with a ventricular peritoneal shunt (VPS) underwent a MRI. Which of the following tests should be done before and after the MRI?
    a. Transcranial dopplers.
    b. CT scan of the head.
    c. Skull series.
    d. Tinetti scores.

82. Which of the following is not an indicator of an anoxic brain injury in adults?
    a. Bradycardia.
    b. Decorticate posturing.
    c. Babinski reflex.
    d. Fixed pupils.

83. A patient diagnosed with acute disseminating encephalomyelitis (ADEM) is placed on high dose steroids. Which of the following should be closely monitored?
    a. Creatinine.
    b. Glucose.
    c. Troponin.
    d. Lactate.

84. Which of the following transmission routes poses the highest risk of contracting Creutzfeldt-Jakob disease (CJD)?
    a. Sexual transmission.
    b. Respiratory droplet.
    c. Exposure to spinal cord fluid.
    d. Blood transfusion.

85. Which of the following most likely cause of cerebrovascular accidents in young patients?
    a. Marijuana.
    b. Alcohol.
    c. Tobacco.
    d. Cocaine.

86. A female patient was admitted to the hospital for stroke. She has a known history of sickle cell disease and tobacco abuse. Her vital signs and lab studies are as follows: BP 126/69, EKG shows normal sinus rhythm, HA1c is 5.2%, Na 145, K 4.1, Cl 100, CO2 30, BUN 19, Cr 1.2, glucose 106, LDL 95, HDL 58, cholesterol 151, beta HCG 8,500mIU/mL, WBC 10.1, hemoglobin 12.4, hematocrit 38.5, platelets 258,000. How many risk factors did this patient have for developing a stroke?
   a. One.
   b. Two.
   c. Three.
   d. Four.

87. A patient arrives at the hospital status post assault with altered mental status. Her eyes open to noxious stimuli, she makes inappropriate responses to questions, and she is moving spontaneously, but is not following commands. Which of the following most accurately describes her Glasgow Coma Scale (GCS)?
   a. E3V4M6.
   b. E2V4M5.
   c. E3V3M5.
   d. E2V3M5.

88. A patient has been admitted for new onset seizures. During her hospital stay she is diagnosed with glioblastoma multiform. She refuses tell her husband who is inquiring about the patient's diagnosis. Which of the following the next appropriate step? (Select all that may apply).
   a. Have the patient's primary care doctor tell the husband.
   b. Give the husband a copy of the radiology reports.
   c. Tell the husband in private.
   d. Request that the husband speak to his wife.

89. Which of the following signs and symptoms does NOT occur in both Parkinson's disease and Huntington's disease?
   a. Chorea.
   b. Tremor.
   c. Ataxia.
   d. Muscle rigidity.

90. A patient is brought to the hospital status post assault to the head with a blunt object. The patient opens his eyes to verbal commands, withdraws to noxious stimuli, and is making incomprehensible verbal responses. Which of the following Glasgow Coma Score (GCS) is correct regarding the patient's verbal ability?
   a. One.
   b. Two.
   c. Three.
   d. Four.

91. An infant arrives in the emergency room obtunded. The mother states that the baby fell off of a couch onto the floor. On physical exam the baby has bilateral retinal hemorrhages and hemotympanum. On CT of the head without contrast the patient has bilateral hypodense concavities. Which of the following is the most appropriate management? (Select all that may apply).
    a. Division of Youth and Family Services (DYFS) referral.
    b. 1:1 observation.
    c. Neurosurgery consult.
    d. Call the police.

92. A patient presents to the emergency room with a severe headache. A CT of the head is negative. An aneurismal subarachnoid hemorrhage is suspected and the patient undergoes a lumbar puncture. Which is true regarding the number of red blood cells in the first bottle of cerebrospinal fluid (CSF) compared to the fourth bottle?
    a. The number of red blood cells stays the same.
    b. The number of red blood cells goes up.
    c. The number of red blood cells goes down.
    d. There is no set pattern.

93. Which of the following is not a therapeutic intervention for patients in vasospasm due to an aneurysmal subarachnoid hemorrhage?
    a. Hypertension.
    b. Hemodilution.
    c. Hyperventilation.
    d. Hypervolemia.

94. Which of the following illustrates the classic triad seen in Parkinson's disease?
    a. Hypokinesia, chorea, dementia.
    b. Ataxia, urinary incontinence, dementia.
    c. Ascending muscle weakness, paresthesias, dysphagia.
    d. Hypokinesia, resting tremor, rigidity.

95. What is a common complication seen with a temporal bone fracture?
    a. Chronic headaches.
    b. Meningitis.
    c. Cerebrospinal fluid (CSF) leak.
    d. Paralysis.

96. A male patient was admitted to the hospital for stroke. He has a known history of cocaine use. His vital signs and lab studies are as follows: BP 201/89, EKG shows atrial fibrillation with 110 bpm, HA1c is 5.6%, complete blood count and basic metabolic panel are unremarkable. How many risk factors did this patient have for developing a stroke?
    a. One.
    b. Two.
    c. Three.
    d. Four.

97. Which of the following signs is not part of Cushing's triad?
    a. Unequal pupils.
    b. Hypertension.
    c. Bradycardia.
    d. Irregular respirations.

98. What is the primary etiology of Pfeiffer Syndrome?
    a. Development of cleft palate.
    b. Hemifacial atrophy.
    c. Underdevelopment of facial nerves.
    d. Premature fusion of cranial sutures.

99. A patient status post motor vehicle accident is diagnosed with an 8 mm right parietal epidural hematoma. The patient had lost consciousness following the accident. Currently the patient's Glasgow Coma Scale (GCS) is fifteen. Which of the following is most appropriate intervention?
    a. Discharge home.
    b. Surgical evacuation.
    c. Obtain serial imaging.
    d. External ventricular drain.

100. Which of the following statements regarding schwannomas are true? (Select all that may apply).
    a. They are slow growing tumors.
    b. Schwannomas may cause hearing loss.
    c. They are more common in females.
    d. Tobacco abuse is a risk factor.

101. Which of the following areas is the primary center for fine motor control?
    a. Occipital lobe.
    b. Cerebellum.
    c. Brainstem.
    d. Frontal lobe.

102. Which of the following would be affected in a frontal lobe tumor? (Select all that may apply).
    a. Personality.
    b. Writing.
    c. Language comprehension.
    d. Judgment.

103. A patient with a history of seizures just suffered an acute seizure. Her family member states that she takes phenytoin (Dilantin) for her condition. Her Dilantin level is 6.1μg/mL. Which of the following labs should be ordered when ordering a Dilantin level to monitor therapy?
    a. Albumin.
    b. Sodium.
    c. Chloride.
    d. Prolactin.

104. A patient presents to the office with worsening generalized headache for several weeks. He also mentions that his hands and feet have become larger over the past several years; his gloves and shoes no longer fit. On physical exam he has a prominent jaw and forehead as well as enlarged lips, nose, and tongue. Which of the following may be the reason for his symptoms?
   a. Pineal tumor.
   b. Craniopharyngioma.
   c. Pituitary adenoma.
   d. Astrocytoma.

105. A trauma patient arrives in the emergency room making few incomprehensible sounds, withdrawing to pain, and opening eyes to verbal command. Which of the following scores is correct in regards to the verbal assessment?
   a. Two.
   b. Three.
   c. Four.
   d. Five.

106. All of the following is true regarding Tourette's syndrome except?
   a. It is characterized by voluntary vocalizations or movements.
   b. There is no standard treatment regimen.
   c. It affects males more commonly than females.
   d. Onset usually occurs in childhood.

107. A 26-year-old female with a known history of alcohol abuse is admitted for gastroenteritis. She clinically improves and is discharged home. Several weeks later she returns to the hospital and is diagnosed with Guillain-Barré syndrome (GBS). How many risk factors does she have for GBS?
   a. One.
   b. Two.
   c. Three.
   d. Four.

108. Which of the following is a risk factor for cerebral palsy (CP)? (Check all that may apply).
   a. Meconium aspiration
   b. TORCH infections
   c. Hyperglycemia
   d. Normal spontaneous vaginal delivery

109. Which of the following is not a treatment for tension headaches?
   a. Tramadol (Ultram).
   b. Ibuprofen (Motrin).
   c. Sumatriptan (Imitrex).
   d. Levetiracetam (Keppra).

110. A patient presents with intermittent headaches associated with nausea and vomiting for the past several months. The headaches usually occur with the onset of menses. Prior to the onset of symptoms she describes seeing strange lights. Which of the following is the most likely diagnosis?
   a. Meningitis.
   b. Migraine headaches.
   c. Meniere's disease.
   d. Multiple sclerosis.

111. Which of the following signs and symptoms are most consistent with Meniere's disease?
    a. Vertigo, headache, vision loss.
    b. Headache, dizziness, nausea.
    c. Vertigo, hearing loss, tinnitus.
    d. Fever, neck pain, headache.

112. What is the most common cause of gigantism in pediatric patients?
    a. Astrocytoma.
    b. Pineocytoma.
    c. Choriocarcinoma.
    d. Pituitary adenoma.

113. What is the most common complication of an intraventricular hemorrhage (IVH)?
    a. Seizure.
    b. Hydrocephalus.
    c. Cortical blindness.
    d. Paralysis.

114. A 56-year-old female is brought to the hospital following an assault to the head. A CT of the head reveals an indeterminate hypodensity. A CT angiogram of the brain reveals a 16mm middle cerebral artery aneurysm. Which of the following is the most appropriate intervention?
    a. Surgical repair.
    b. Discharge home.
    c. Serial imaging as an outpatient.
    d. Lumbar puncture.

115. A patient fell off of a ladder landing on his buttocks three hours ago arrives in the emergency room complaining of worsening back and lower extremity paresthesias. Which of the following questions is the most important initial question?
    a. Do you have any medical problems?
    b. Have you any changes in your bowel or urinary habits?
    c. When did your symptoms start?
    d. Do you have a power of attorney?

116. Where do medulloblastomas most commonly occur?
    a. Pons.
    b. Spinal cord.
    c. Brain stem.
    d. Cerebellum.

117. A patient with known history of chronic alcohol abuse is brought to the emergency room for withdrawal symptoms. In the ER he develops a seizure. Once a seizure ends, another begins several minutes later. Which of the following is the most appropriate initial action?
    a. Order a banana bag.
    b. Administer phenytoin (Dilantin).
    c. Prepare for intubation.
    d. Obtain a CT of the head.

118. Which of the following regarding medulloblastomas is true?
    a. They most commonly occur in pediatric patients.
    b. Maternal drug use is a significant risk factor.
    c. Radiation is a common treatment modality.
    d. They are usually benign.

119. A patient is diagnosed with cauda equine syndrome. What is the mainstay of treatment for this condition?
    a. Plasmapheresis.
    b. Pain medications.
    c. Surgery.
    d. Steroids.

120. Which of the following medications is primarily given for status epilepticus?
    a. Pentobarbital (Nembutal).
    b. Phenytoin (Dilantin).
    c. Levetiracetam (Keppra).
    d. Lorazepam (Ativan).

121. Which of the following is not consistent with Brown-Sequard syndrome?
    a. Loss of sensation on the ipsilateral side of the injury.
    b. Loss of pain on the contralateral side of the injury.
    c. Loss of temperature on the contralateral side of the injury.
    d. Loss of movement on the ipsilateral side of the injury.

122. Which of the following are signs and symptoms are indicative of a skull fracture? (Select all that may apply).
    a. Visual changes.
    b. Battle sign.
    c. CSF leak from the ears.
    d. Raccoon eyes.

123. A patient who has a history of a cerebrovascular accident one year ago suffers another stroke. The patient's only past medical history are obesity and poorly controlled diabetes. The patient takes aspirin (Ecotrin) as an outpatient. Which of the following medications should be added? (Select all that may apply).
    a. Clopidogrel (Plavix).
    b. Warfarin (Coumadin).
    c. Atorvastatin (Lipitor).
    d. Amiodarone (Cordarone).

124. What is a potential common side effect of intravenous phenytoin (Dilantin) administration?
    a. Tardive dyskinesia.
    b. Pruritus.
    c. Hypotension.
    d. Bowel incontinence.

125. A patient is admitted for an acute ischemic stroke. His wife asks why his blood pressure is allowed to run higher than usual. Which of the following is the most appropriate response?
    a. Hypertension will increase perfusion to the ischemic areas of the brain.
    b. Hypertension decreases the risk of a hemorrhagic stroke.
    c. Hypertension may help prevent against seizures.
    d. Hypertension may reverse some of the damage caused by the stroke.

126. A patient arrives to emergency room with symptoms of a possible stroke. Which of the following is the most important initial question to ask?
    a. Have you ever had a stroke?
    b. What time did the symptoms start?
    c. Do you have any past medical history?
    d. What medications do you take?

127. A patient with a confirmed right-sided ischemic stroke is receiving tissue plasminogen activator (tPA) when she suddenly develops a right-sided hemiparesis. What is the most appropriate intervention?
    a. Send the patient for CT head.
    b. Discontinue the tPA.
    c. Administer aspirin/Ecotrin.
    d. Obtain an electroencephalogram (EEG).

128. Which of the following patients have the lowest risk for stroke?
    a. 56-year-old man with a history of atrial fibrillation.
    b. 68-year-old woman with a HA1C of 6.2%.
    c. 25-year-old woman with a history of cocaine abuse.
    d. 37-year-old patient in sickle cell crisis.

129. Which of the following terms means difficulty speaking and understanding speech?
    a. Apnea.
    b. Ataxia.
    c. Aphasia.
    d. Dyslexia.

130. Diagnostic tests for non-infectious etiology of epilepsy include all of the following EXCEPT:
    a. blood cultures.
    b. electroencephalogram (EEG).
    c. CT of the head.
    d. Wada test.

131. All of the following statements about Lou Gehrig's disease are true EXCEPT:
    a. it causes degeneration and death of upper and lower motor neurons.
    b. patients lose strength and control of voluntary muscles.
    c. it progresses rapidly and is fatal.
    d. it impairs cognition and senses.

132. Which of the following is true regarding Bell's palsy? (Select all that may apply).
   a. Facial droop may be a presenting sign.
   b. No actual permanent damage occurs.
   c. It is a harbinger of a future stroke.
   d. A virus may precipitate the onset of symptoms.

133. Which type of seizure may be mistaken for attention deficient hyperactivity disorder (ADHD)?
   a. Simple complex seizure.
   b. Grand mal seizure.
   c. Petit mal seizure.
   d. Pseudoseizure.

134. AIDS increases the likelihood of developing which of the following? (Select all that may apply).
   a. Meningitis.
   b. Dementia.
   c. Encephalitis.
   d. Central nervous system lymphomas.

135. What are the three signs and symptoms that characterize posterior reversible encephalopathy syndrome (PRES)?
   a. Bradykinesia, tremor, muscle rigidity.
   b. Dysphagia, ascending weakness, respiratory distress.
   c. Fever, vomiting, neck pain.
   d. Headache, seizures and visual loss.

136. A patient is admitted to the hospital for altered mental status and subsequently diagnosed with diagnosed with posterior reversible encephalopathy syndrome (PRES). The patient's daughter asks about the prognosis of her father's condition. Which of the following is the most appropriate response?
   a. The prognosis is good and residual deficits are unlikely.
   b. The prognosis is good, but residual deficits are common.
   c. The prognosis is guarded and residual deficits are likely.
   d. The prognosis is poor and withdrawal of care should be considered.

137. A patient admitted to the hospital with altered mental status and fever is subsequently diagnosed with Cryptococcus meningitis. What other test should be ordered for this patient? (Select all that may apply).
   a. Western blot.
   b. Blood cultures.
   c. CD4/CD8 count.
   d. Enzyme-linked immunosorbent assay (ELISA).

138. A patient recently diagnosed with multiple sclerosis (MS) asks how it is caused. Which of the following is the most appropriate response?
   a. It is caused by destruction of the myelin sheath of nerve cells.
   b. It is caused by the destruction of the substantia nigra.
   c. It is cause by an immune mediated response to peripheral neurons.
   d. It is caused by an additional copy of chromosome 21.

139. What is the most common course of multiple sclerosis (MS)?
    a. Secondary progressive.
    b. Primary progressive.
    c. Relapsing remitting.
    d. Progressive relapsing.

140. Which of the following may cause seizures? (Select all that may apply).
    a. Heroin.
    b. Methamphetamines.
    c. Cocaine.
    d. Oxycodone (Oxycontin).

141. Which of the following may cause a seizure? (Select all that may apply).
    a. Alcohol.
    b. Meningitis.
    c. Cocaine.
    d. Subdural hematoma.

142. A patient presents with moderate receptive aphasia, severe expressive aphasia, and left-sided weakness. The patient is subsequently diagnosed with glioblastoma multiforme (GBM). Where is this lesion most likely located?
    a. Left temporal lobe.
    b. Left frontal lobe.
    c. Right temporal lobe.
    d. Right frontal lobe.

143. Which of the following is a leading neurological cause of death in the U.S.A.?
    a. Cerebrovascular accident.
    b. Malginancy.
    c. Epidural hematoma.
    d. Status epilepticus.

144. A mother brings her son to the emergency room for recurrent seizures. She states that he developed seizures early in his childhood. The episodes include tonic-clonic movement involving the neck, shoulders, upper arms, and face. What type of seizure is this child experiencing?
    a. Petite mal.
    b. Simple partial.
    c. Tonic clonic.
    d. Myoclonic.

145. Which of the following are true regarding ependymoma? (Check all that apply).
    a. It is more common in children than in adults.
    b. The location is commonly intracranial in adult patients.
    c. The location is commonly spinal in pediatric patients.
    d. The primary treatment is chemotherapy.

146. A 69-year-old male has fallen and lost consciousness. He has a laceration on his head and is breathing very rapidly. Which of the following may be in the differential diagnosis? (Select all that may apply).
    a. Seizure.
    b. Mechanical fall.
    c. Stroke.
    d. Drug overdose.

147. A patient presents with a sudden right facial droop and dysarthria. Which of the following would like likely be in the differential diagnosis? (Select all that apply).
    a. Meningitis.
    b. Bell's palsy.
    c. Cerebrovascular accident.
    d. Malignancy.

148. Which of the following is not a treatment for atonic seizures?
    a. Dietary modifications.
    b. Callosotomy.
    c. Haloperidol (Haldol).
    d. Vagus nerve stimulator.

149. A patient arrives in the emergency room status post motorcycle accident. His Glasgow Coma Scale (GCS) is thirteen. The patient has facial lacerations, a cephalohematoma, clear fluid pooling in his ear, and weakness in his bilateral lower extremities associated with incontinence. Which of these issues should be addressed first?
    a. Cephalohematoma.
    b. Fluid in his ear.
    c. Facial lacerations.
    d. Extremity weakness and incontinence.

150. Which of the following is not a sign or a symptom of a pituitary microadenoma?
    a. Increased serum prolactin level.
    b. Increased bone density.
    c. Infertility.
    d. Galactorrhea.

151. A patient arrives in the emergency room with altered mental status. Which of the following would be the initial part of the evaluation?
    a. Order a neurosurgery consult.
    b. Obtain a blood glucose level.
    c. Order a CT of the head.
    d. Obtain an electroencephalogram (EEG).

152. A patient status post motor vehicle accident suffered a depressed skull fracture. The emergency physician notes that the patient is having Cheyne–Stokes respirations. Which of the following best describes this breathing pattern?
    a. Irregular respirations.
    b. Rapid respirations.
    c. Shallow respirations.
    d. Slow deep breaths.

153. What is shock caused by injury to the spinal cord called?
    a. Hypovolemic.
    b. Undifferentiated.
    c. Neurogenic.
    d. Obstructive.

154. An adult male has been shot in the neck. He is awake and alert with palpable upper and lower extremity pulses. There is a small wound to the right lateral side of his neck, with minor bleeding. Which of the following best describes the sequence of care?
    a. Leave the wound open and have the patient remain supine.
    b. Cover the wound with an occlusive dressing and have the patient remain supine.
    c. Leave the wound open and have the patient remain sitting.
    d. Cover the wound with an occlusive dressing and have the patient remain sitting.

155. How long can brain cells survive if circulation ceases?
    a. 1-2 minutes.
    b. 3-4 minutes.
    c. 5-6 minutes.
    d. 8 –10 minutes.

156. What substance do damaged neurons secrete that initiates the destructive cascade of apoptosis?
    a. Hydrogen peroxide.
    b. Carbon dioxide.
    c. Glutamate.
    d. Epinephrine.

157. When do most deaths following a middle cerebral artery (MCA) occlusion generally occur?
    a. 1-2 days.
    b. 3-4 days.
    c. 5-6 days.
    d. 7-10 days.

158. Restoring circulation to the ischemic penumbra can limit brain damage in an ischemic infarct. How long is this window of opportunity following the onset of symptoms?
    a. 1-2 hours.
    b. 3-4 hours.
    c. 5-6 hours.
    d. 7-10 hours.

159. Which of the following is the most likely negative outcome of a basilar artery fusiform aneurysm?
    a. Infarct.
    b. Seizure.
    c. Subarachnoid hemorrhage.
    d. Negative outcome is unlikely.

160. Which of the following sequelae is not caused by an intracranial aneurysm? (Select all that may apply).
    a. Seizure.
    b. Permanent neurological deficit.
    c. Subarachnoid hemorrhage.
    d. Hydrocephalus.

161. A patient with a C4 fracture status post diving accident is being admitted to the intensive care unit. Which of the following is the most important initial assessment?
    a. Administer an electrocardiogram.
    b. Insert a foley catheter.
    c. Check capillary refill of upper and lower extremities.
    d. Assess oxygenation status and respiratory rate.

162. A 76-year-old patient who woke up with left hemiparesis came to the emergency room within one hour of waking up. She is diagnosed with an acute right middle cerebral artery (MCA) stroke and admitted to the hospital. Her husband wants her to receive tissue plasminogen activator (tPA) because they arrived at the hospital within one hour of discovering the symptoms. Which of the following is the most appropriate explanation why she did not receive tPA?
    a. TPA can't be given when the time of onset of symptoms is unknown.
    b. TPA increases the risk of cerebral hemorrhage in elderly patients.
    c. TPA cannot be given to those with MCA strokes.
    d. TPA is not given to those with severe symptoms such as hemiparesis.

163. A patient who had suffered a large acute stroke needs to be fed. Which of the following is the most appropriate management?
    a. Obtain a speech evaluation prior to feeding.
    b. Allow the patient to rest comfortably in the supine position.
    c. Offer the patient pureed food.
    d. Suction the patient's secretions between bites of food.

164. Which of the following patients should be assessed first?
    a. 23-year-old with a migraine headache who is complaining of severe nausea and vomiting.
    b. 45-year-old who is scheduled for a craniotomy in 30 minutes.
    c. 59-year-old with Parkinson's disease who needs a swallowing assessment.
    d. 63-year-old with a recent stroke and worsening dysarthria.

165. A patient admitted to the hospital with an acute right-sided ischemic stroke is being evaluated in the intensive care unit. Which of the following would be the most concerning for the medical team?
    a. The blood glucose level is 303 mg/dL.
    b. Patient failed his swallow evaluation.
    c. Patient is no longer able to lift his left arm.
    d. The patient's blood pressure is 159/88.

# Answers and Explanations

1. C: The patient's phenytoin (Dilantin) level is supratherapeutic. A normal level is 10-20 mcg/mL. Supratherapeutic levels can cause confusion, nausea, urticaria, nystagmus, hypotension, and cardiac arrhythmias. Naloxone/Narcan can reverse narcotic medications, but not phenytoin. Holding the medication and checking serial levels is the mainstay of management.

2. B: A patent foramen ovale (PFO) is a hole between the left and right atria of the heart. It normally closes shortly after birth. This condition may cause the formation of clots which can travel to the brain leading to a transient ischemic attack or stroke. In the event that this happens a patient may need to be placed on antiplatelet medications or blood thinners. The other factors are risk factors for thrombotic stroke.

3. D: Antiepileptic drugs are not indicated for subacute hemorrhagic brain injuries. The greatest risk of seizure is in the first two weeks following the incident. If no seizure has occurred during this time then antiepileptic drugs do not need to be prescribed for the patient.

4. A: Astrocytomas arise from astrocytes, which are a type of glial cell; they are the most common glial tumor. Surgical resection in conjunction with chemotherapy and radiation are common treatments. Grades I and II are generally benign slow growing tumors seen in children, whereas grades III and IV are malignant and typically seen in adults.

5. D: The overwhelming majority of ALS cases are idiopathic. This neuromuscular degenerative disease occurs at random with no clearly associated risk factors. Individuals with this sporadic form of the disease do not have a family history of ALS, and their family members are not considered to be at increased risk for developing it. In a small majority of cases occur with a family history of this disease. Multiple gene mutations are involved with developing this condition.

6. A: Cluster headaches occur due to an unknown etiology. They are characterized by unilateral symptoms that may involve the eye on the ipsilateral side. Treatment includes triptan drugs, calcium channel blockers, and steroids.

7. C: Neurofibromatosis occurs due to a genetic defect, which causes tumors to arise from nerve cells. Complications that may occur from this disorder include deafness, hypertension, seizures, hydrocephalus, scoliosis, pathologic fractures, kyphosis, and vision problems. Common signs and symptoms include light brown spots on the skin called café-au-lait spots, abnormal development of the spine, skull, or long bones, freckling in the area of the armpit or the groin, and disturbances in balance.

8. B: This condition describes type II, which is the most common type of Chiari malformation. Type I is where the lower part of the cerebellum, but not the brainstem extends into the foramen magnum. Type III is where part of the cerebellum and the brainstem extend through the foramen magnum into the spinal cord causing severe neurologic impairment. Chiari malformation type IV is not associated with herniation of the brain through the foramen magnum; it involves an underdeveloped cerebellum. This type is usually fatal in infancy.

9. D: The signs and symptoms of Chiari malformation can vary greatly from one person to another. The most common associated symptom is occipital headache caused by the herniation of the brain

through the skull base. Other signs and symptoms include diplopia, nystagmus, visual changes, and balance difficulties.

10. A: Administering D50 would be appropriate since the patient's glucose is 43, which may be the reason for the altered mental status and dysarthria. If the patient's neurological exam doesn't improve once the blood sugar normalizes, then obtaining a CT of the head would be appropriate. If the CT of the head is negative then administering tPA would be the next step if there are no contraindications. The patient's GCS is 12; not sufficiently low enough to warrant intubation.

11. A: Multiple sclerosis (MS) is a chronic progressive autoimmune disease that attacks the myelin sheath of nerve cells. It can occur at any point in life but is most common in the third and fifth decades of life. It can affect either sex, but affects women more than men. There is no cure but immunosuppressive medications, muscle relaxers, and steroids may help with symptomatic relief of acute flare-ups. For unknown reasons it is more common to people indigenous to temperate climates such as the United States and Europe.

12. C: Fibromyalgia is a medical condition with unknown etiology characterized by chronic pain. Other signs and symptoms may include dysphagia, sleep disturbances, and bowel and bladder disturbances. Labs and imaging studies are normal. This condition is often associated with depression and anxiety. There a wide range of treatments for this disorder including anti-depressant and anti-anxiety medications, lifestyle changes to limit stress, bowel regimens, elimination of gluten, acupuncture, and sleep aids.

13. B: Initial treatment for this patient would be conservative management. The patient may ambulate with physical therapy wearing an LSO brace. She may take pain medications and receive steroid injections for symptomatic relief. If repeat imaging in several weeks shows instability of the fracture or the patient has intractable pain then surgical intervention may be considered.

14. D: GBS doesn't cause brain abscesses. GBS is an autoimmune disease that causes damage to the body's peripheral nerves causing rapid onset weakness, dysphagia, and respiratory difficulties. This condition may be treated with plasmapheresis and high dose steroids. Any immunocompromised state such as AIDS or malignancy can predispose a person to infection. Injuries that can introduce pathogens to the brain such as calvarial (skull) fractures, facial fractures, sinusitis or dental infections may predispose a patient to developing a brain abscess.

15. D: Obtaining an EEG is the most appropriate step since the patient recently had a seizure. The patient is postictal, but is still following commands so intubation at this point is not warranted. TPA is contraindicated in those who present with a seizure. Intracranial hemorrhage, recent head trauma in the last three months, active internal bleeding, uncontrolled blood pressure (>185/100), abnormal clotting factors due to malignancy or anticoagulation (INR > 1.7, platelet count <100,000), glucose <50 mg/dL or > 400 mg/dL, and seizure at stroke onset are other absolute contraindications to tPA. Discharging the patient is inappropriate; the patient needs a neurology consult, serial neurological exams, further stroke work-up, and an EEG prior to discharge home.

16. B, C: TGN affects the trigeminal or 5th cranial nerve. TGN is caused by compression or damage to the nerve. It may also be associated with multiple sclerosis, which damages the myelin sheath of nerve cells. There are a variety of treatments used for TGN, which include anticonvulsant medications, steroids, NSAIDs, narcotic pain medications, and surgery. TGN commonly affects women more than men. Flare-ups commonly occur during the day during periods of activity like chewing, coughing, or talking.

17. A, B, C: Garbanzo beans, collard greens, and oranges are excellent sources of folate. Garlic is not a significant source of folic acid. A major risk factor for developing spina bifida is a mother with a folate deficiency. All women who are trying to conceive should take a folate supplement (800 mcg) to help prevent their fetus from developing spina bifida.

18. A: This patient's signs and symptoms are consistent with postherpetic neuralgia. Once infected with varicella (chickenpox) the virus remains latent in the central nervous system. It may become reactivated later during periods of stress, illness, or immunosuppression. Anti-inflammatory medications, narcotic analgesics, and lidocaine patches may provide some symptomatic relief.

19. C: The patient's GCS is seven; E2V1M4.

# Glasgow Coma Scale

| | | |
|---|---|---|
| Best eye response (E) | Spontaneous--open with blinking at baseline | 4 |
| | Opens to verbal command, speech, or shout | 3 |
| | Opens to pain, not applied to face | 2 |
| | None | 1 |
| Best verbal response (V) | Oriented | 5 |
| | Confused conversation, but able to answer questions | 4 |
| | Inappropriate responses, words discernible | 3 |
| | Incomprehensible speech | 2 |
| | None | 1 |
| Best motor response (M) | Obeys commands for movement | 6 |
| | Purposeful movement to painful stimulus | 5 |
| | Withdraws from pain | 4 |
| | Abnormal (spastic) flexion, decorticate posture | 3 |
| | Extensor (rigid) response, decerebrate posture | 2 |
| | None | 1 |

20. B: The patient likely has a herniated disc. An abscess or a tumor should be ruled out since the pain is alleviated with rest and the patient has no other associated signs or symptoms. Meningitis typically presents with neck pain, fever, chills, seizure, and lethargy.

21. B: Compression on the median nerve which controls sensation and motor ability in the first, second, third, and fourth digits causes carpal tunnel syndrome. Repetitive motion, autoimmune diseases, and pregnancy predispose people to this condition. On physical exam the Phalen's sign may be positive. The medical practitioner may have the patient hold their arms out in front of them and then flex their wrists, letting their hands hang down for about sixty seconds. If numbness and tingling occur, the patient may have carpal tunnel syndrome. Treatment options may include

NSAIDs, rest, ice, wrist splint, and carpal tunnel release surgery for those who fail conservative management.

22. B, C, D: Studies have shown that immobilizing the neck for long periods of time can decrease muscle strength and impair recovery. If a collar is to be worn infrequently for short periods of time. Using NSAIDS as needed, lidocaine injections, and applying ice/heat to the neck several times a day are appropriate recommendations for the treatment of whiplash.

23. A, B, C: The last statement is an inappropriate treatment for a CSF leak. When the volume of CSF becomes low, the brain will sag inside the skull, causing headaches that worsen when the patient is in a sitting or upright position. Being in a supine position minimizes the effects of gravity and alleviates symptoms.

24. D: Haemophilus influenzae (H. flu) is a bacterium that can cause a severe infection, occurring mostly in infants and children younger than five years of age. Vaccines given to children in the first year of life have significantly decreased the incidence of H. flu meningitis. Cryptococcus meningitis is an opportunistic fungal infection primarily seen in immunocompromised patients. Neisseria and Listeria infections are generally seen in older adults.

25. B: There is no evidence of hydrocephalus on the CT scan and an external ventricular drain is not warranted. This patient has an epidural hematoma, which requires emergent surgical evacuation. An antiepileptic drug should be administered prior to the procedure and a week or two following the procedure to decrease the risk of seizure. Serial neurological exams should be performed to monitor the patient's condition. Although their GCS is high, many patient with epidural hematomas present with a lucid interval and then rapidly decompensate. The mortality rates of these types of injuries are high and aggressive treatment is needed.

26. B, D: BPPV is caused by a problem in the inner ear. Calcium deposits inside your inner ear canals help maintain one's balance. Infections or inflammation can stop the stones from moving as they should. This sends a false message to the brain and causes the vertigo. BPPV is a recurrent condition. There is no one specific treatment for BPPV; however there are several options to help prevent future flare-up. Different body positions/exercises, sleeping on the unaffected side, increasing one's fluid intake, antihistamines, and sedatives may help treat and prevent symptoms.

27. A, B: Intracranial hemorrhage, recent head trauma in the last three months, active internal bleeding, uncontrolled blood pressure (greater than 185/100), abnormal clotting factors due to malignancy or anticoagulation (INR greater than 1.7, platelet count less than 100,000), glucose less than 50 mg/dL or greater than 400 mg/dL, and seizure at stroke onset are other absolute contraindications to tPA.

28. A: Cushing's triad is defined as irregular respirations, bradycardia, and hypertension. It is a physiologic nervous system response to persistent increased intracranial pressure (ICP). Normal intracranial pressures measure <20mmHg. Persistent elevated ICPs in addition to the appearance of Cushing's triad is a sign of impending herniation.

29. C: The physical exam finding describes a positive Brudzinski sign, which is seen in those with meningitis. This is caused by the inflammation surrounding the brain and spinal cord.

30. B, D: The classic NPH triad includes dementia, urinary incontinence, and ataxia.

31. C: Meniere's disease is a chronic progressive disease due to a disorder of the inner ear. It causes periodic vertigo, tinnitus, nausea, vomiting, and ultimately permanent loss of hearing. The condition is not fatal. The etiology is believed to be multifactorial. Since hearing is affected, a referral to an audiologist is the most appropriate intervention.

32. D: The patient has Pott's disease or spinal tuberculosis. Tuberculosis may originate in the lungs and spread to the spine or the primary infection may be in the spine. In this patient's case, he had pulmonary tuberculosis approximately one year ago, which went untreated, and then spread to his spine. It is more common in third world countries. Non-immunocompromised patients with have a positive purified protein derivative (PPD). Depending on the amount of bony destruction and severity of symptoms treatment may be conservative (anti-TB medications, bracing, and pain medications) or surgical intervention.

33. C: Her motor exam would be scored as a six. Her eye response is a two and her verbal response is a five. Her total GCS score is thirteen.

# Glasgow Coma Scale

| | | |
|---|---|---|
| Best eye response (E) | Spontaneous--open with blinking at baseline | 4 |
| | Opens to verbal command, speech, or shout | 3 |
| | Opens to pain, not applied to face | 2 |
| | None | 1 |
| Best verbal response (V) | Oriented | 5 |
| | Confused conversation, but able to answer questions | 4 |
| | Inappropriate responses, words discernible | 3 |
| | Incomprehensible speech | 2 |
| | None | 1 |
| Best motor response (M) | Obeys commands for movement | 6 |
| | Purposeful movement to painful stimulus | 5 |
| | Withdraws from pain | 4 |
| | Abnormal (spastic) flexion, decorticate posture | 3 |
| | Extensor (rigid) response, decerebrate posture | 2 |
| | None | 1 |

34. B: Triple-H therapy (hypervolemia, hemodilution, and hypertension) aim to increase cerebral perfusion in aneurysmal subarachnoid hemorrhage and help prevent vasospasm. Calcium channel blockers cause dilatation of the vasculature. IV fluids cause hemodilution. Vasopressors cause permissive hypertension while the patient is in the vasospasm window, which lasts approximately two weeks. Diuretics prevent hemodilution and may cause hypotension and hypovolemia; therefore, they are not utilized.

35. A: The patient likely suffered a stroke in the vertebrobasilar area, which controls balance, gait and vision. Although patients may present with a variety of signs and symptoms, drop attacks are common findings with those who have vertebrobasilar strokes.

36. B: Hydrocephalus is a possible complication of a BGB. The blood may obstruct outflow of cerebrospinal fluid requiring an external ventricular drain and possibly a ventricular peritoneal shunt. Blindness or visual changes would be seen in pathology of the occipital cortex. Hearing may be damaged if trauma or pathology occurred to the temporal bone or inner ear. Seizures are unlikely to occur as a result from trauma or pathology of deep brain structures.

37. D: Supplementation with thiamine, as well as other electrolytes such as magnesium and potassium is important in treating WKS. WKS typically presents with the classic triad of confusion, ataxia, and nystagmus commonly seen in chronic alcoholic patients.

38. A, B: AVMs are rare conditions that involve abnormal connections of veins and arteries that usually occur in the brain and spine. The cause of brain AVM is unknown, but most believe most brain AVMs emerge during fetal development. There is no known genetic inheritance. Not all AVMs need surgical resection. Some may be corrected with endovascular embolization or Cyber-Knife. If the patient is a poor surgical candidate, if the patient is asymptomatic, or the AVM was an incidental finding, serial imaging may be done to monitor it.

39. C: DAI is caused by shearing of the small blood vessels in the brain following an assault or high speed collision. CT scans may miss the findings associated with DAI. MRIs are the test of choice since they are more sensitive. A hypodense convexity best describes an epidural hematoma. Choice 'b' describes findings associated with hydrocephalus. A hypodense concavity describes a subdural hematoma.

40. C: The patient has five risk factors: male sex, advanced age, hyperlipidemia, diabetes, and hypertension. As people become older their risk of stroke increases. Males tend to have strokes more often than females. His LDL and cholesterol are high and his HDL or "good" cholesterol is low (see chart below). A nondiabetic patient will have a hemoglobin A1c less than 5.7%. A hemoglobin A1c between 5.8-6.2% is a borderline diabetic; it may resolve with lifestyle modifications and diet. If the HA1c is above 6.2% the patient should be placed on oral anti-hyperglycemic medication(s). The goal HA1c in diabetic patients is <less than7.0%. The patient's blood pressure is also incredibly high which may have contributed to his stroke (see chart below).

LDL

| <100 | Optimal |
|---|---|
| 100-129 | Near Optimal |
| 130-159 | Borderline High |
| 160-189 | High |
| ≥190 | Very high |

Total Cholesterol

| <200 | Desirable |
|------|-----------|
| 200-239 | Borderline High |
| ≥240 | High |

HDL Cholesterol

| <40 | Low |
|-----|-----|
| ≥60 | High |

Blood Pressure

| <120/80 | Optimal |
|---------|---------|
| 120-139/80-89 | Prehypertension |
| 140-149/90-99 | Stage I hypertension |
| >150/100 | Stage II hypertension |

41. A: The occipital lobes house the primary vision centers so visual change or acute vision loss is a common finding in acute occipital lobe strokes. Posterior headaches are another common finding.

42. A: Surgical removal of half a dozen bilateral brain lesions is not possible. If there was one particularly large lesion that was felt to be the primary cause of symptoms and the lesion was in an accessible location, surgical debulking may be attempted. However, in this patient's case, whole brain radiation therapy, anticonvulsant drugs, and steroid therapy would be the mainstays of treatment.

43. B, C, D: All of the interventions except for the first option are reasonable management measures. A 16-year-old female with a history of depression and no risk factors for seizure is suspect for having pseudoseizure. A pseudoseizure is an intentional or unintentional psychosomatic physical manifestation of stress or anxiety. It is nonepileptic in nature. It is seen most often in pre-pubescent and teenage females.

44. D: Radiation therapy is the most common treatment modality for spinal tumors. However surgery and bracing is the second most common. Most spinal tumors are the result of metastatic disease. Prostate, lung, and breast cancer frequently spreads to the bone. Bony metastases are usually associated with a poorer prognosis.

45. B: Compression on the median nerve which controls sensation and motor ability in the first, second, third, and fourth digits causes carpal tunnel syndrome. Repetitive motion, autoimmune diseases, and pregnancy predispose people to this condition. On physical exam the Phalen's sign may be positive. The medical practitioner may have the patient hold their arms out in front of them and then flex their wrists, letting their hands hang down for about sixty seconds. If numbness and tingling occur, the patient may have carpal tunnel syndrome.

46. B: The Dix-Hallpike maneuver is a classic diagnostic test for BPPV. The patient starts in sitting position on exam table facing forward with their eyes open. The examiner rapidly lies patient backward and turns the patient's head to the right with the neck extended hanging over end of table. The examiner has the patient rapidly sit back up and then repeats the maneuver with the patient's head facing toward the left. If rapid repositioning causes vertigo, but the patient is asymptomatic at rest, then the patient is diagnosed with BPPV.

47. A, D: WKS is due to a thiamine deficiency commonly seen in chronic alcoholic patients although it can occur in those with dietary deficiencies in thiamine (Beriberi). The classic triad is ocular disturbances (opthalmoplegia), ataxia, and dementia.

48. C: A patient with a nondepressed skull fracture who is neurologically intact can follow up as an outpatient as long as the attending felt that the patient would be compliant with follow up. No surgical intervention is warranted.

49. B: Oligodendrogliomas are indolent malignant primary brain tumors that are generally responsive to chemotherapy. Patients may live ten years or more after the initial onset of symptoms.

50. A: Chemotherapy and radiation are the most effective treatments for germinomas. Germinomas are the most common type of malignant pineal tumor. The pineal gland controls the various bio-rhythms of the body. It helps regulate circadian rhythms by secreting melatonin as well as regulation of reproductive hormones. The cause of pineal malignancies is largely unknown. Signs and symptoms of malignancy include hydrocephalus, seizure, memory disturbances, and visual disturbances. Prognosis is very good with early aggressive treatment.

51. D: Oligodendromas are slow growing tumors that most commonly occur in the frontal and temporal lobes. The most common signs and symptoms are headaches, seizures, and personality changes. The etiology of these types of tumors is unknown. They are typically treated with surgical resection, chemotherapy, and radiation.

52. A: The patient likely has a traumatic brain injury and a CT of the head needs to be obtained. The patient's Glascow Coma Scale (GCS) is an eleven. He should be admitted to an intensive care unit for close monitoring, but does not need to be intubated at this time. The general rule for GCS is "less than eight-intubate." There is no mention of seizure or agitation so antiepileptic drugs and restraints would be inappropriate measures.

# Glasgow Coma Scale

| | | |
|---|---|---|
| Best eye response (E) | Spontaneous--open with blinking at baseline | 4 |
| | Opens to verbal command, speech, or shout | 3 |
| | Opens to pain, not applied to face | 2 |
| | None | 1 |
| Best verbal response (V) | Oriented | 5 |
| | Confused conversation, but able to answer questions | 4 |
| | Inappropriate responses, words discernible | 3 |
| | Incomprehensible speech | 2 |
| | None | 1 |
| Best motor response (M) | Obeys commands for movement | 6 |
| | Purposeful movement to painful stimulus | 5 |
| | Withdraws from pain | 4 |
| | Abnormal (spastic) flexion, decorticate posture | 3 |
| | Extensor (rigid) response, decerebrate posture | 2 |
| | None | 1 |

53. B: The patient's aneurysm is relatively small and will need to be monitored as an outpatient. Smoking, uncontrolled hypertension, vascular disorders such as Marfan's Syndrome, and genetics are common causes of aneurysms. The patient's family will likely not need to be scanned since the patient has several risk factors for developing an aneurysm. Aneurysms occur in a small percentage of the population and any time one is found it will require follow up. Urgent surgical intervention is indicated for aneurysms greater than 6 mm.

54. C, D: CT angiogram and transcranial dopplers (TCDs) are the best tests used to detect vasospasm. TCDs are used more routinely since they do not involve dye and have much less radiation.

55. B: Vasospasm is a feared complication of those with ruptured aneurysms because it can lead to further brain injury. The highest risk for vasospasm occurs 14-21 days after the onset of the bleed. It can occur earlier or later than this time period, but the risk drops significantly.

56. C: Chondrosarcomas are rare tumors that occur on the sphenoid bone which frequently cause headaches and visual changes. Surgical resection is the mainstay of treatment. The etiology of this condition is unknown.

57. A: Unilateral tinnitus and hearing loss are the most common presenting symptoms of a person with a schwannoma. Schwannomas are slow growing benign tumors of the acoustic nerve. The etiology is unknown. Surgical resection is the mainstay of treatment.

58. A, B, C, D: All of the treatments listed would be appropriate for treating a child with cerebral palsy. There is not one correct treatment; treatment must be tailored to the severity and type of symptoms. Antiepileptic drugs, muscle relaxants, dopaminergic drugs, Botox, as well as non-pharmacologic therapies such as physical, occupational, and speech therapies may minimize symptoms and maximize quality of life.

59. D: Parkinson's is a progressive neurodegenerative disease where the substantia nigra is slowly destroyed. The substantia nigra produces dopamine. Classic signs and symptoms of Parkinson's include shuffling gait, mask-like facies, rigidity, micrographia, and resting tremor.

60. C: Folate deficiency is the primary reason for development of spina bifida. Most medical practitioners recommend 800 mcg of folate per day while trying to conceive. Taking a folate supplement after conceiving will not help prevent spina bifida since the neural tube has already formed.

61. C: This patient has essential tremor. It usually occurs in the 4-6th decades of life and improves with rest, but worsens with activity. In contrast, Parkinson's tremor improves with activity and is most noticeable with rest. Simple motors seizures are not affected by activity. Tourette's syndrome is characterized by involuntary tics or noises, which are not affected by activity.

62. A: Although any cancer can spread to the brain, gastrointestinal malignancies have a smaller likelihood of doing so. The most common malignancies to metastasize to the brain are breast and lung cancer as well as malignant melanoma.

63. B: Meningitis can be caused by fungi, viruses or bacteria and is passed through contact and respiratory droplets. It spreads quickly in those who live in close quarters such as college dormitories, prisons, and army barracks.

64. A, C, D: All of the interventions are correct except placement of a urinary catheter. Unless the patient has urinary retention or an obstruction, there is no reason to place a foley catheter in a stroke patient. Indwelling catheters increase patients' risk for infection.

65. A: Tremor is the most common movement disorder. The exact etiology for essential tremor is not known, but it is more likely to occur in those who have family members with this condition. Treatment of essential tremor usually begins with primidone (Mysoline) or propranolol (Inderal) monotherapy.

66. A: Petit mal or absence seizures generally involve short periods of spontaneously resolving blank staring episodes most commonly seen in children ages 4-14 years of age.

67. A: Febrile seizures may occur in children as young as three months old to six years of age. The earlier a child has a febrile seizure, the higher likelihood that they will have another in the future.

Anticonvulsant therapy is typically not used in the treatment of febrile seizures. Febrile seizures tend to run in families. There is minimal risk of neurologic impairment unless the patient suffers significant head trauma during the seizure.

68. D: Brainstem strokes affect functions that are essential for life such as heart rate, temperature control, swallowing, and blood pressure. Language comprehension and formation are affected with pathology of the temporal lobe.

69. B: Vascular disorders such as Marfan's syndrome, tobacco abuse, hypertension, and atherosclerosis are common causes of carotid dissection. Sometimes it may be due to an idiopathic cause. However, trauma to the neck is the most common reason for it to occur in young people. The treatment is the same no matter the etiology; people are treated with anticoagulation and antiplatelet regimens. Angioplasty is usually offered to those where anticoagulation is contraindicated.

70. C: Chronic uncontrolled hypertension is the most common cause for basal ganglia and thalamic bleeds. Since these areas are deep in the brain, surgical evacuation is generally not performed. However if the blood extends into the ventricles, hydrocephalus may develop warranting external ventricular drain placement.

71. A, B, D: Exercise is not a known trigger for seizures. Common trigger may include hypoglycemia, significant dehydration, stress, alcohol, sleep deprivation, head trauma, and severe illness.

72. B: The mother had toxoplasmosis and passed it to her unborn child. Toxoplasmosis is one of the TORCH viruses (Toxoplasmosis, Other, Rubella, Cytomegalovirus, and Herpes) which commonly cause fetal anomalies. Wild and domestic felines are the parasite's predominant hosts. Contact with infected feces, water bowls, or food trays can transmit the parasite to the mother with mild effects. However the parasite can have devastating effects on the unborn fetus such as hearing loss, developmental delays, blindness, and hydrocephalus requiring shunting.

73. B: Memory is primary controlled in the frontal and temporal lobes. The parietal lobe is responsible for reading, writing, calculations, and sensations.

74. A: In order to prevent the risk of developing a spinal headache, patients should lie flat, refrain from alcoholic beverages, increase their fluid intake, and be on light duty/activity 24-48 hours following the procedure.

75. C: Epilepsy is defined as two more seizures that occur in a twenty-four hour period with no preceding cause (i.e. trauma, overdose, illness).

76. A: Fetal Alcohol Syndrome is the leading cause of preventable physical and mental fetal abnormalities. It presents with a variety of signs and symptoms but the classic triad is smooth philtrum, thin vermilion border, and microcephaly. Other signs and symptoms include impaired fine motor skills, neurosensory hearing loss, poor gait, clumsiness, poor impulse control, impaired communication, difficulty with math, and growth retardation.

77. D: Pellagra presents with the classic triad dermatitis, dementia, and diarrhea. Other signs and symptoms include ataxia, paralysis, and peripheral neuritis. It is due to simple dietary lack of niacin (vitamin B3), which can be found in meat, poultry, fish, eggs, and peanuts.

78. D: Anencephaly is a condition in which the neural tube forms improperly and major parts of the brain fail to develop. Fetuses who survive with this condition are born without cerebral hemispheres, which govern thinking and coordination of movement. These babies usually don't live past infancy.

79. B: Herpes simplex II is one of the TORCH viruses (Toxoplasmosis, Other, Rubella, Cytomegalovirus, and Herpes), which commonly cause fetal anomalies. Common signs and symptoms include lethargy, irritability, tremor, poor feeding, temperature instability, and full anterior fontanelle.

80. A, B, D: All of the modalities are appropriate except for bedrest. Alzheimer patients should be encouraged to exercise to help maintain mobility. Frequent rest breaks should be offered to prevent fatigue and falls.

81. C: Skull series are s special type of x-rays that should be taken before and after a MRI to confirm that the VPS dial has not shifted position. Transcranial dopplers are used to evaluate vasospasm in aneurysmal subarachnoid hemorrhages. CT scans do not evaluate the position of the VPS dial. Tinetti scores are used to measure ataxia and have no role in evaluating VPS placement.

82. A: Bradycardia may be present in those with anoxic brain injuries, but is not a sign of brain injury. Signs and symptoms of anoxic brain injury may include no flow on a brain flow study, lack of respirations with ventilator support, loss of corneal or gag reflexes, decorticate posturing, abnormal reflexes such as the appearance of the Babinski reflex in adults, fixed pupils, and persistent vegetative state without underlying cause (i.e. hypothermia).

83. B: Patients on steroids need to be monitored for hyperglycemia, hypokalemia, and sleep disturbances. There may be mood changes (irritability, crying, anxiety) when people are on steroid therapy. Other reversible complications of steroid therapy include weight gain, flushed cheeks, and facial swelling.

84. C: The risk of spreading CJD is low. It is spread through contact of infected brain tissue or spinal fluid. Sporadic CJD is not spread through airborne droplets, blood, or sexual contact. CJD is a transmissible spongiform encephalopathy that causes rapid neurological deterioration. There is no treatment and the condition is always fatal.

85. D: Cocaine is a common cause of strokes in young patients. Tobacco and alcohol are risk factors for stroke, but generally need to be chronically abused over long periods of time. Cocaine can cause a stroke shortly after being used. Urine drug screens should be administered to all young patients who suffer can ischemic stroke that do not have any underlying risk factors (i.e. sickle cell disease).

86. C: The patient has three risk factors for stroke. She has sickle cell disease, she uses tobacco products, and she is pregnant. Her beta HCG is 8,500mIU/mL. A normal beta HCG in nonpregnant females is 5mIU/mL. Pregnancy is a hypercoagulable state and can predispose those with existing underlying factors to developing a cerebrovascular accident.

87. D: The patient's Glasgow Coma Scale is ten. Her verbal response is given two points, her verbal response is given three points, and her motor exam is given five points.

# Glasgow Coma Scale

| | | |
|---|---|---|
| Best eye response (E) | Spontaneous--open with blinking at baseline | 4 |
| | Opens to verbal command, speech, or shout | 3 |
| | Opens to pain, not applied to face | 2 |
| | None | 1 |
| Best verbal response (V) | Oriented | 5 |
| | Confused conversation, but able to answer questions | 4 |
| | Inappropriate responses, words discernible | 3 |
| | Incomprehensible speech | 2 |
| | None | 1 |
| Best motor response (M) | Obeys commands for movement | 6 |
| | Purposeful movement to painful stimulus | 5 |
| | Withdraws from pain | 4 |
| | Abnormal (spastic) flexion, decorticate posture | 3 |
| | Extensor (rigid) response, decerebrate posture | 2 |
| | None | 1 |

88. D: Due to HIPAA (Health Insurance Portability and Accountability Act) a medical practitioner may not disclose medical information to anyone without the patient's consent. The patient is likely in denial about her diagnosis and would benefit from grief counseling or a psychiatrist evaluation.

89. A: Chorea is involuntary writhing movements that are seen in Huntington's disease and not in Parkinson's disease. Parkinson's disease is a progressive neurodegenerative disorder that presents classically with bradykinesia, micrographia, mask-like facies, muscle rigidity, resting tremor, and ataxia. It is due to the destruction of the substantia nigra which produces dopamine. Huntington's disease is an autosomal dominant neurodegenerative disorder that presents with tremor, ataxia, chorea, mania, muscle rigidity, and seizure.

90. B: The patient's verbal ability is a two according to the GCS. Being oriented is five points, confused is four points, inappropriate is three points, incomprehensible is two points, and no verbal response is one point.

91. A, B, C: Calling the police is not warranted. Referring the case to DYFS is sufficient since they can turn into criminal investigations. A 1:1 observation in the child's room can help monitor suspicious activity when visitors are present. A neurosurgery referral is needed to monitor and possibly evacuate the patient's subdural hematomas. Hemotympanum is usually seen with severe blunt

force trauma and retinal hemorrhages are generally seen when young children are shaken violently. A fall off a couch does not explain the child's injuries.

92. A: One way to diagnose an occult aneurysmal subarachnoid hemorrhage is to do a lumbar puncture and draw four bottles of CSF. In subarachnoid hemorrhages, the blood doesn't clear and the number of red blood cells present is essentially the same in the first and fourth bottle. In traumatic lumbar punctures the number of red blood cells decreases with each successive tube drawn.

93. C: Triple H therapy for subarachnoid hemorrhages include induced hypertension through fluid boluses or vasopressors, hemodilution through aggressive IV fluid hydration, and hypervolemia through blood transfusions help treat vasospasm.

94. D: Hypokinesia, resting tremor, and muscle rigidity are the classic symptoms. However, Parkinson's can also include with mask-like facies, erectile dysfunction, micrographia, dementia, and postural instability.

95. C: A CSF leak from the ear canal is a common occurrence in temporal bone fractures since it houses many of the auditory structures. Meningitis may occur but it is not a common complication. Chronic headaches and paralysis are not complications of temporal bone fractures.

96. D: Male sex, cocaine use, hypertension, and atrial fibrillation are all risk factors for stroke. Other risk factors can include pregnancy, hyperlipidemia, diabetes, coronary artery disease, obesity, and tobacco abuse.

97. A: Cushing's triad or reflex is seen with impending cerebral herniation. The classic symptoms include irregular respirations, bradycardia, and hypertension. Fixed pupils may be seen with herniation, but is not part of this clinical trial.

98. D: Pfeiffer Syndrome is a chromosomal disorder that results in the premature fusion of cranial sutures. It causes bulging eyes and an underdeveloped midface. There are usually no associated cognitive deficits.

99. B: Surgical evacuation is the most appropriate intervention for an epidural hematoma. They are extra-axial bleeds almost exclusively seen with high impact trauma. They may present with a lucid interval before patients develop neurological symptoms. Approximately twenty percent of epidural hemorrhages are fatal. The primary treatment is surgical evacuation.

100. A, C: The first and third statements are correct. Schwannomas are slow growing tumors that affect the seventh cranial nerve. They are more common in females. Surgery is the primary treatment. They may cause facial paralysis, dysphagia, abnormal eye movements, and ataxia.

101. B: The cerebellum is responsible for fine motor movements as well as balance and coordination.

102. A, D: The frontal lobe controls personality, judgment, decision-making ability, inhibition, planning, mood, and reasoning ability. Writing is primarily controlled by the parietal lobe and language comprehension is controlled by the temporal lobe.

103. A: Dilantin levels should always be corrected for albumin. Since most of the Dilantin in serum is bound to proteins, the level of serum albumin influences the amount of free Dilantin.

104. C: The patient has the physical findings of acromegaly, which is caused by pituitary adenomas in adults. The pituitary secretes growth hormone (GH); since the growth plates in adults have already fused, thickening of the bones and enlargement of the hands and feet occur. Surgery is the first option recommended for most people with acromegaly.

105. A: The patient's verbal assessment would be scored as a two. The patient's Glasgow Coma Scale (GCS) is nine; E3V2M4.

# Glasgow Coma Scale

| | | |
|---|---|---|
| Best eye response (E) | Spontaneous--open with blinking at baseline | 4 |
| | Opens to verbal command, speech, or shout | 3 |
| | Opens to pain, not applied to face | 2 |
| | None | 1 |
| Best verbal response (V) | Oriented | 5 |
| | Confused conversation, but able to answer questions | 4 |
| | Inappropriate responses, words discernible | 3 |
| | Incomprehensible speech | 2 |
| | None | 1 |
| Best motor response (M) | Obeys commands for movement | 6 |
| | Purposeful movement to painful stimulus | 5 |
| | Withdraws from pain | 4 |
| | Abnormal (spastic) flexion, decorticate posture | 3 |
| | Extensor (rigid) response, decerebrate posture | 2 |
| | None | 1 |

106. A: Tourette's syndrome is characterized by <u>involuntary</u> vocalizations or movements. There is no known cause. Onset usually occurs in childhood and improves by early adulthood. It affects males more commonly than females. There is no standard treatment regimen. Antipsychotic medications such as Haloperidol/Haldol may be used to help suppress symptoms.

107. A: Guillain-Barré syndrome (GBS) is an autoimmune disorder in which the body attacks the peripheral nervous system. It presents as ascending paresthesias and weakness which may vary in severity. There is no known cause, but upper respiratory infections, gastrointestinal infections, surgery, and vaccinations, particularly the influenza vaccination may increase the risk for developing GBS. GBS occurs in all age groups and affects both sexes equally. This patient has one risk factor which is her recent gastroenteritis.

108. A, B: The first two statements are risk factors for CP. CP is a neurological disorder that affects cognition, muscle tone and strength, and coordination. Other risk factors include low birth weight, a delivery requiring the use of instruments or an emergency Caesarean section, birth asphyxia, postnatal seizures, and hypoglycemia.

109. D: Anticonvulsants such as Keppra are not used in the treatment for tension headaches. Narcotics, triptans, NSAIDs, anticonvulsants, and muscle relaxers are common remedies.

110. B: This patient has the classic symptoms of a migraine headache. Migraines are chronic severe headaches that may be preceded by prodromal symptoms such as altered vision, sound, or taste call an aura.

111. C: Meniere's disease is caused by excessive fluid in the inner ear causing vertigo, tinnitus, and progressive hearing loss. Other signs and symptoms may include, nausea, vomiting, diaphoresis, and drop attacks. Treatment modalities include diuretics, reduction of sodium intake, antihistamines, and stress reduction therapies such as yoga or meditation.

112. D: Pituitary adenomas cause gigantism in children due to the overproduction of growth factor. Since children's growth plates have not closed is causes uncontrolled growth. In adults pituitary adenomas cause acromegaly.

113. B: Hydrocephalus is a common complication in IVH due to the obstruction of outflow of cerebrospinal fluid (CSF). Bleeds that occur deep in the brain typically do not cause seizures. Pathology in the occipital lobes may cause vision impairment. Paralysis may occur with IVH depending on the size of the bleed, but hydrocephalus is more common.

114. A: Unruptured cerebral aneurysms larger than 6 mm require surgical intervention since they have a high risk of bleeding. Ruptured aneurysms no matter the size require surgery. Small unruptured aneurysms less than 3-4 mm can be followed as an outpatient with serial imaging. Unruptured aneurysms that are 5-6 mm can be monitored closely as an outpatient if the patient is a poor surgical candidate.

115. B: Urinary or bowel retention or incontinence in conjunction with a history of fall and back pain may indicate a significant spinal abnormality. A potential complication of this patient's injury is cauda equina syndrome, which would require urgent surgical decompression.

116. D: Medulloblastomas most commonly occur in the cerebellum. They are rare malignancies that most commonly occur in children.

117. B: The patient is in status epilepticus and needs to be intubated. Status epilepticus is when a seizure begins without recovery from a prior seizure. The most important initial intervention is to secure the patient's airway. Medications may be administered while the patient is being intubated. A CT of the head is appropriate once the patient is safely intubated.

118. A: Medulloblastomas are rare malignant tumors. They are the most common pediatric brain malignancy. Primary treatments are chemotherapy and surgical debulking. Radiation is not an option due to most patients' young age. The exact cause is unknown.

119. C: Cauda equina syndrome requires emergent surgical decompression. The cauda equine is a collection of nerve roots between the conus medullaris and the filum terminale. Damage, usually

- 89 -

due to a traumatic event such as a fall, can cause saddle anesthesias, urinary/bowel incontinence or retention, back pain, rectal pain, and lower extremity paresthesias. If left untreated patients may progress to permanent paralysis and permanent urogenital dysfunction. Steroids may be given to alleviate swelling, but surgical intervention is the only definitive treatment.

120. A: Pentobarbital is a short acting barbiturate used in the treatment of status epilepticus that has failed benzodiazepine and traditional anticonvulsant therapy.

121. D: In patients with Brown Sequard syndrome the sensory loss is particularly strong on the ipsilateral side as the injury to the spine. These sensations are accompanied by a loss of the sense of pain and of temperature on the contralateral side at which the injury was sustained.

122. A, B, C, D: All of the following choices may indicate a skull fracture. Raccoon eyes (periorbital ecchymoses) and Battle sign (ecchymoses behind the ears) can be the result of a basilar skull fracture. A CSF leak may occur with a temporal bone fracture; a patient may note CSF coming from their ears or nose. Visual changes may occur with posterior skull fractures since they may affect the occipital lobes. Other signs and symptoms of skull fractures include nausea, vomiting, headache, seizures, and change in pupil size.

123. A, B: Since the patient already had a stroke a second antiplatelet agent such as Plavix should be added. Lipitor should also be added to reduce the risk of future thromboembolic events. Coumadin and/or Amiodarone would be considered if the patient had a history of atrial fibrillation, patent foramen ovale, or a mechanical valve.

124. C: Hypotension is a serious common side effect of IV Dilantin. If a patient is being given IV Dilantin they should be on a telemetry monitor to closely assess vital signs. If there is a mild drop in blood pressure a fluid bolus should be given. However, if a significant drop occurs of if the patient develops symptoms, the drug should be discontinued.

125. A: Permissive hypertension following the first few days of a stroke may increase perfusion to ischemic parts of the brain limiting the damage of the stroke. Hypertension does not reverse damage by the part of the brain involved in a stroke. Dead brain cells cannot be revived. Hypertension must be carefully monitored because if the blood pressure rises too high it increases the risk of developing a hemorrhagic stroke. Hypertension does not prevent seizures.

126. B: Finding out the time of onset of the symptoms will determine whether or not the patient is eligible for tissue plasminogen activator (tPA). Newest guidelines recommend that tPA may be given up to 4.5 hours after symptom onset as long as the patient does not have any major contraindications.

127. B: The most important initial step is to discontinue the tPA. One of the most feared complications of tPA is development of a cerebral hemorrhage. Since the patient has a confirmed right stroke, the patient should have left-sided symptoms. Since the patient has right-sided hemiparesis, left brain pathology is suspected. The medical team should discontinue tPA and then get a CT head of the patient. If that is negative then an EEG may be considered. Antiepileptic drugs should be held off unless the EEG is positive or seizure is strongly suspected.

128. B: The elderly female with borderline diabetes has the lowest incidence of stroke. Although diabetes increases risk for stroke, her diabetes is well controlled. A nondiabetic patient will have a hemoglobin A1c less than 5.7%. A hemoglobin A1c between 5.8-6.2% is a borderline diabetic; it

may resolve with lifestyle modifications and diet. If the HA1c is above 6.2% the patient should be placed on oral anti-hyperglycemic medication(s). The goal HA1c in diabetic patients is < 7.0%. Atrial fibrillation, cocaine abuse, and sickle cell disease significantly increase the risk for stroke.

129. C: Aphasia is the impaired ability to form and understand speech. Receptive aphasia is in inability to understand speech. Expressive aphasia is the inability to form speech. Global aphasia is a combination of both. Aphasia is usually due to damage of the temporal lobe.

130. A: Blood cultures are not typically part of epilepsy work-up unless an infectious source is suspected. EEGs help detect current or recent seizure activity, CT head will help detect a structural abnormality (i.e. tumor) that may be causing the seizure activity, and the Wada test is used to determine which side of the brain controls language and memory function. It is generally ordered if an epilepsy patient is considering surgery.

131. D: ALS, also known as Lou Gehrig's disease, is a rapidly progressive, fatal neurological disease that attacks the upper and lower nerve cells responsible for controlling voluntary muscles. It does not affect cognition or affect a person's ability to see, smell, taste, hear, or recognize touch. There are no known risk factors for the disease. Goals of therapy are to keep the patient mobile and independent for as long as possible.

132. A, D: Bell's palsy is unilateral paralysis or weakness of the facial muscles due to damage to the facial nerve. The weakness may or may not be permanent depending on the damage. It does not signal an eventual future stroke. The cause is not completely understood, but it is believed to be caused by a recent viral infection.

133. C: Petit mal seizures, also known as absence seizures, involve frequent staring episodes followed by a postictal period. These seizures are typically seen in children. Due to the atypical presentation they may be mistaken for ADHD.

134. A, B, C, D: AIDS gradually destroys the immune system, which makes patients vulnerable to developing opportunistic bacteria, fungi, and viruses resulting in encephalitis and meningitis. AIDS dementia complex (ADC) occurs primarily in persons with more advanced HIV infection. CNS lymphomas are almost always associated with the Epstein-Barr virus. Prognosis is poor due to advanced and increasing immunodeficiency.

135. D: PRES is characterized by headache, confusion, seizures, and visual loss. Deficits are usually not permanent once the underlying cause is treated. Etiologies may include malignant hypertension and eclampsia.

136. A: The prognosis for PRES is generally good. Patients with PRES develop cerebral edema due to a reversible etiology such as malignant hypertension. The goal is to treat the underlying cause. Deficits are usually not permanent once the underlying cause is successfully treated.

137. A, B, C, D: All of the following may be ordered for this patient. The ELISA test is the first initial test to diagnose a patient with AIDS and the Western blot is the confirmatory test. The CD4/CD8 count is the measurement of special types of lymphocytes that help battle infection in the body. This test may help direct treatment in a patient with HIV/AIDS. Blood cultures may be ordered to evaluate if an underlying septicemia is present.

138. A: MS is caused by the idiopathic destruction of the myelin sheath of nerve cells affecting coordination, balance, sensation, vision, and motor strength. It is a progressive neurological disease with no known cause or cure. Goal of care is to minimize exacerbations and maximize quality of life.

139. C: The most common disease course of multiple sclerosis is relapsing remitting. People with this type have intermittent flares followed by full, partial, or no recovery. Primary progressive and secondary progressive MS are less common. Primary progressive MS is where the patient steadily declines without plateau or remission. Secondary progressive is where the patient originally has relapsing remitting but then steadily declines without plateau or remission. Progressive relapsing MS is the least common form of the disease. Symptoms steadily get worse, but people also have intermittent flares.

140. B, C: Opiates such as heroin and Oxycodone do not cause or exacerbate seizure activity. They may cause other complications such as depressed central nervous system function, addiction, and death.

141. A, B, C, D: All of these options may cause seizures. Other etiologies may include structural deformities such as Chiari malformation, brain lesions such as tumors, and brain surgery.

142. C: The GBM is most likely located in the right temporal lobe which houses the brain's main language processing centers. Since the brain has contralateral control of the body, the lesion will be on the right side if the patient is experiencing left-sided weakness.

143. A: CVAs are the leading neurological cause of death in the United States. Other leading causes include heart disease, cancer, and accidents. CVAs are the leading cause of serious, long-term disability.

144. D: The child is having myoclonic seizures. Myoclonic seizures usually cause abnormal movements on both sides of the body at the same time involving the neck, shoulders, upper arms, and face. The onset usually occurs in childhood or around puberty. In most cases these seizures can be well controlled with medication, but these medications but be taken for the patient's entire life.

145. A: Ependymomas are more common in children and usually are located in the posterior fossa in pediatric patients. The primary treatment is surgical debulking.

146. A, B, C, D: All of these could be reasons why the man had fallen. A CT of the head and a MRI of the brain should be obtained along with vascular studies of the head and neck, electroencephalogram, and a urine drug screen should be ordered. In addition orthostatics, a 2D echo, troponins, fingerstick, urinalysis, and a physical therapy evaluation should be ordered to further assess the patient.

147. B, C: Bell's palsy and stroke are the most likely diagnoses. Meningitis typically presents with headache, fever, nuchal rigidity, altered mental status, and seizure. Malignancies usually involve a gradual progressive worsening of symptoms.

148. C: Haldol is not used in the treatment of atonic seizures also known as drop seizures. In drop seizures muscles suddenly lose strength and the person may drop things and often falls to the ground. Atonic seizures usually begin in childhood. Surgery, vagus nerve stimulators, and antiepileptic drugs are the mainstays of treatment. Several studies have shown that the ketogenic diet helps prevent seizures in children whose seizures could not be controlled by medications.

149. D: The patient likely has a significant spinal cord injury and cauda equine needs to be ruled out. The patient needs to be kept on bedrest with serial neurological exams until emergent imaging of the spine and neurosurgical referral can be obtained. The patient likely has a concussion and possibly an intracranial bleed with a likely skull fracture, but since the GCS is relatively high, these issues can be addressed second.

150. B: Decreased bone mineral density may be seen with pituitary microadenomas. Observation or surgery may be considered as treatment depending on the severity of symptoms and size of the tumor. Medications such as bromocriptine may also be used.

151. B: Hypoglycemia is a common cause of confusion and should be ordered prior to ordering more expensive and invasive tests and procedures.

152. A: Cheyne–Stokes breathing involves irregular respirations with intermittent periods of apnea. It can be seen in patients with significant trauma where the brain's respiratory center is damages, immature neonates, those who venture into high altitude locations, and patients with heart failure.

153. C: Neurogenic shock is a type of shock that causes decreased systemic vascular resistance caused by damage to the autonomic pathways in the spine. Patient may develop severe hypotension and may go into respiratory and/or cardiac arrest.

154. D: Open wounds to the neck have to be occluded immediately to reduce the chance of air leaking into the neck tissue or into a lacerated artery or vein that may cause a possible air embolus. Having the patient sit up instead of remaining supine prevents the risk of aspiration.

155. A: Brain cells are incredibly sensitive to oxygen deprivation and will survive for about 1-2 minutes once circulation ceases.

156. C: Injured neurons discharge glutamate, which acts on the damaged neurons adjacent ones initiating a destructive cascade.

157. B: Deaths due to MCA infarctions generally occur due to cerebral edema, which usually doesn't fully develop until the third or fourth day following the event.

158. B: The opportunity to give tissue plasminogen activator (tPA) is up to 4.5 hours following symptom onset. The earlier tPA is given the greater the chance of limiting the amount of brain damage. Giving tPA after this time period will likely have minimal chance of limiting neurological deficit, but greatly increases the risk of cerebral hemorrhage.

159. A: Fusiform aneurysms of the basilar artery usually undergo thrombosis causing ischemic infarction of the pons. Subarachnoid hemorrhage due to rupture and seizure are uncommon occurrences.

160. A, B, C, D: All of the options may be caused by an aneurysm. If it ruptures it may cause hydrocephalus, subarachnoid hemorrhage, seizure, permanent neurological deficit, and death.

161. D: Assessing the patient's respiratory status is of utmost importance due to the high level of spinal injury. Patients with cervical spine trauma office develop respiratory insufficiency or distress and need to be monitored closely.

162. A: While the patient did manage to arrive in the hospital within one hour of waking up, the exact time of onset of symptoms is unknown because she woke up with left hemiparesis. After 4.5 hours tPA should not be given since it significantly increases the risk of a cerebral hemorrhage and does not significantly improve the brain damage that has already occurred.

163. A: Any patient with an intracranial injury should have a speech evaluation performed to assess their swallowing ability. A speech pathologist may recommend a modified diet, which will decrease the likelihood of aspiration.

164. D: Any patient with a recent stroke with a new neurological change needs a stat CT of the head or MRI of the brain to evaluate for hemorrhage and/or cerebral edema. The other patients' needs are important, but are not life threatening.

165. C: Any patient with a recent stroke with a new neurological change needs a stat CT of the head or MRI of the brain to evaluate for hemorrhage and/or cerebral edema. The other issues are important, but are not life threatening.